Lucas Fontana Tomasini

Using tools to monitor dairy cattle herds

Lucas Fontana Tomasini

Using tools to monitor dairy cattle herds

Evaluation of faeces score, locomotion score, trough score, body condition score and rumen score

ScienciaScripts

Imprint

Any brand names and product names mentioned in this book are subject to trademark, brand or patent protection and are trademarks or registered trademarks of their respective holders. The use of brand names, product names, common names, trade names, product descriptions etc. even without a particular marking in this work is in no way to be construed to mean that such names may be regarded as unrestricted in respect of trademark and brand protection legislation and could thus be used by anyone.

Cover image: www.ingimage.com

This book is a translation from the original published under ISBN 978-613-9-69269-9.

Publisher:
Sciencia Scripts
is a trademark of
Dodo Books Indian Ocean Ltd. and OmniScriptum S.R.L publishing group

120 High Road, East Finchley, London, N2 9ED, United Kingdom
Str. Armeneasca 28/1, office 1, Chisinau MD-2012, Republic of Moldova, Europe
Printed at: see last page
ISBN: 978-620-8-12965-1

ACKNOWLEDGEMENTS

Firstly, I thank God for the strength that always helps me achieve my goals.

I would like to thank all my family, especially my mother for all the effort she put into my studies, for her teachings and help at all times, my stepfather who is undoubtedly my real father, my grandparents who helped me a lot in my life and always gave me a lot of strength during university.

To my girlfriend, who I love very much, for all the times she was by my side helping me, for the moments of joy and difficulty.

To my university classmates and friends, for all the moments we experienced, especially Clério, Odinei, Lagoa, Tafa, Bola, Bocão, Hornero, Henrique, Ismael, Anderson, Dani, Suian, Andreia and Perna, Jéssica, Lilian, Zamoner, JP, Carminatti, Mario, Lucas Huf, Lucas Brehm. Also the other class I studied with and will be graduating with, Xuxa, Naibo, Sherlon, Ansilieiro, Forti, Cristian, Luiz, Rafa, Neuri, Jessica, Gabi, Bárbara, Cândida, Piolho, Aline, Renata.

I would like to thank all the teachers, especially Professor Luis Fabiano, "Rochinha", "Juca" and Paulo Bennemann, for all their help, companionship, friendship and advice, which helped me grow professionally and personally.

I'd like to thank the staff at Nutre, where I did my final internship, especially supervisors Abílio, Marcelo and Frankarlo, for all their learning and trust, and their families for their welcome and lunches.

I would like to thank the entire UNOESC community for the support that has helped my training.

*"**The only** dicde place of succession is the dictionary. " (Albert Einstein)*

SUMMARY

Dairy farming is one of the most widely practised rural activities in our country and is of great social and economic importance. Milk has great nutritional value and is part of our lives. However, in order for the milk to reach the consumer's table with quality, a great deal of work by the Veterinarian, in the field with the producers, is necessary. The curricular internship was carried out at the company NUTRE - Saúde e produção animal, in the city of São **Jorge D'oeste** - PR, from 2 March to 2 May 2015, totalling 360 hours. The activities carried out during the internship were in the areas of preventive medicine, reproductive clinic, medical clinic and property management. The end-of-course work highlights some of the means of monitoring dairy cattle herds: locomotion score, faeces score, body condition score, trough score and rumen score. The scores were assessed on the properties that were part of the company's technical assistance, describing some of the cases encountered and the appropriate procedure. It can be seen that the scores are essential tools for monitoring dairy herds and help to detect errors or management failures, mainly related to nutrition.

Keywords: Dairy cattle. Cattle monitoring. Technical assistance.

SUMMARY

CHAPTER 1

INTRODUCTION

1.1 BACKGROUND

Dairy farming has always been an excellent income option for rural families. In recent years this sector has gone from strength to strength as milk consumption and prices have risen, attracting major investments in infrastructure, genetic improvement and milk quality.

According to the Brazilian Institute of Geography and Statistics (IBGE) (2015), 6.528 billion litres of milk were purchased by milk processors in the fourth quarter of 2014, down 0.2% on the fourth quarter of 2013 and up 4.8% on the third quarter of 2014. Industrialisation, meanwhile, totalled 6.517 billion litres, an increase of 0.1% on the same period in 2013 and 4.8% on the third quarter of 2014.

Along with the sector's growth have come new challenges, where reducing production costs is fundamental to the sustainability of dairy farming. Júnior and Santos (2013), evaluating the growth of national dairy production, pointed out that Brazil is among the world's leading countries, but this position is due to the large number of animals milked and not individual production per animal, indicating that the country still has a lot to invest in the sector with regard to improvements in the areas of management, nutrition and genetics.

The use of tools to monitor dairy herds, which allow problems to be identified through visual assessments, has been growing in recent years. Some examples are the body condition score, the trough score, the faeces score and the locomotion score (SANTOS; CAVALIERI; DAMASCENO, 2002).

The body condition score makes it possible to identify nutritional excesses or deficits. The trough score allows us to identify problems related to the palatability of the diet and factors that affect food consumption, as this is directly related to animal production. The faeces score allows us to identify some nutritional disorders, and can be affected by the dry matter and digestibility of the diet. The locomotion score is a qualitative visual assessment of the cows' ability to walk, which identifies animals with locomotion problems, especially hoof problems. The rumen score helps control feed intake and passage rate (SANTOS; CAVALIERI; DAMASCENO, 2002).

1.2 OBJECTIVES

1.2.1 General objective

The supervised curricular internship aims to assimilate all the knowledge acquired during the academic period with the reality of the field, getting to know the work routine that involves dairy farming, in order to complete the course and train the Veterinarian.

1.2.2 Specific objectives

- Accompanying a veterinarian in the field in dairy farming;
- Monitoring property management;
- Monitoring the technical assistance routine on dairy farms;
- Help diagnose, prevent and treat the main diseases that affect cattle;
- Personal development, in terms of the professional's contact with producers;
- Improve your knowledge of veterinary medicine.

CHAPTER 2

THEORETICAL BACKGROUND

2.1 USING TOOLS TO MONITOR DAIRY CATTLE HERDS

2.1.1   Locomotion score

Hoof and leg diseases are highly prevalent and have a major economic impact on modern dairy farming. The lesions that cause lameness occur in 90% of cases on the hooves of cattle and 10% of lesions occur on the feet. Therefore, prevention and treatment of hoof lesions should be carried out routinely on the farm in order to avoid major losses (OLIVEIRA and SOARES, 2007).

Compared to assessing reproductive performance or udder health, determining the incidence and severity of lameness is a rather subjective task. Lameness in dairy cattle is an economic and welfare issue. According to Juarez et al. (2003), lameness is the third most important economic loss related to animal health in dairy cattle, after fertility and mastitis.

Evaluating the impact of foot alterations on reproductive efficiency in dairy herds, Lee, Ferguson and Galligan (1989) found that cows with clinical lameness before the end of the voluntary waiting period had less frequent oestrus and had longer calving intervals, a longer interval until first service and consequently a longer time until conception. Melendez et al. (2003) carried out a study to analyse the relationship between lameness, ovarian cysts and fertility in dairy cows. They used 65 cows with lameness within 30 days of calving and 130 cows in the control group without lameness. The cows with lameness had a higher incidence of ovarian cysts, 25 per cent, compared to 11 per cent in the control group, and lameness also had an impact on reproduction, as shown in Figure 1.

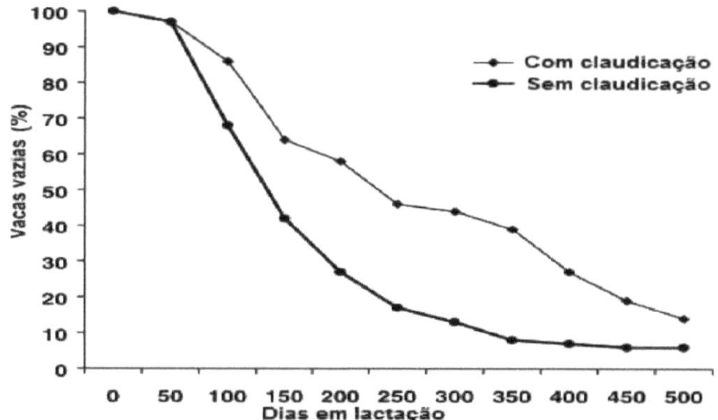

Figure 1 - Comparison of the pregnancy rate between cows with and without lameness.
Source: Melendez et al. (2003).

Warnick et al. (2001), analysing the influence of lameness on milk production on two dairy farms in New York, identified a reduction in daily milk production of between 0.8 and 1.5kg for at least two weeks after the onset of lameness in the cows. The reduction in production was greater in cows with two or more lactations, and the foot diseases that most affected the cows were sole ulcers and hoof abscesses.

Murray et al. (1996) carried out hoof trimming on 37 dairy farms in England and Wales, where they found 8645 lesions associated with lameness. Lesions on the hind limbs accounted for 92 per cent of cases, of which 65 per cent were on the lateral nail, 20 per cent on the skin and 14 per cent on the medial nail. The most common lesions were sole ulcers, white line disease and digital dermatitis. Sulayeman and Fromsa (2012) also studied the prevalence and risk factors of lameness compared to milk production on dairy farms in Ethiopia. A total of 432 cows were assessed and found a prevalence of 3.5 per cent of lameness, of which 2.8 per cent was in the hind limbs. The risk factors found were: pregnancy, nutrition, type of floor, length of rough track, frequency of floor cleaning, age, sex and size of the milking herd.

Dembele et al. (2006) studied factors that contribute to the incidence and prevalence of lameness on some dairy farms in the Czech Republic. The environment of the farms was rated from 1 (excellent) to 5 (very poor) in three different aspects: slippery floors, quality of cow management and the quality of cow care.
quality of the environment. Prevalence ranged from 6% to 42% on the farms visited, where it was found that poorly cared for animals, slippery floors, overgrown hooves, dirty cows and skin lesions are associated with a high prevalence of lameness.

Espejo, Endres and Salfer (2006) studied the prevalence of clinical lameness in 50

Minnesota freestalls. The average prevalence of clinical lameness was 24.6 per cent, which was 3.1 times higher on average than the prevalence estimated by farm employees. They were also able to assess that the prevalence of lameness was lower in freestall herds with sand bedding (17.1 per cent) than in freestall herds with mattress bedding (27.9 per cent). The body condition of the animals was associated with the prevalence of lameness, with animals with body scores below 2.5 having a higher prevalence of lameness (42.57%) than animals with scores between 2.75 and 3.5 (22.05%) and greater than 3.75 (19.68%).

Due to the lack of quantitative measures to assess lameness, most dairy farmers rely on training their staff to determine whether cows are limping or experiencing discomfort when standing or walking. It is usually caused by physical trauma or hoof disease, which will result in increased veterinary costs, increased culling of animals, increased stress, decreased milk production and consequently decreased profitability. Locomotion score systems are useful for assessing the severity, duration and prevalence of lameness (JUAREZ et al., 2003).

The first step in reducing lameness in the herd is to determine the prevalence and severity of lameness. Signs of lameness in dairy cattle include a vertical head bobbing movement when the injured foot makes contact with the ground; arching of the spine associated with pain (cows in extreme discomfort may salivate and grind their teeth); shortening of stride and a reduction in walking speed, with frequent stops to rest the affected limb (NORDLUND et. al., 2004).

All the lactating cows in the herd must be classified. Differences can be observed between lactation groups. According to Nordlund (2004), cows should be scored when walking on a solid, flat surface that is not slippery and is well lit. If repeated observations are made, the same surface should be used. If possible, the herd should be classified by a secondary observer, so that some subjectivity is removed from the classification by having two opinions for discussion. It is interesting that the farm owner or manager is present during or at least for part of the classification process. It is always useful to keep a system of clearly defined records, which should be stored for future analyses.

Using various combinations of these signals, a variety of locomotion score systems have been developed for dairy cattle. There are some practical differences between the systems, but they all have the same intent, to assess how the cows are walking and give a score that will vary from 1-4 or 1-5, depending on the system (SCHLAGETER-TELLO et al., 2014).

2.1.1.1 Locomotion score classification

A locomotion score is a relatively quick and simple qualitative assessment of a cow's ability to walk normally. The gait score, if carried out regularly (e.g. monthly), can be used to identify which cows are at risk of more severe clinical lameness in the future. Group locomotion scores can also be used to estimate financial losses in milk, and the losses can be used as a criterion to determine whether general nutritional or management interventions are necessary (JUAREZ and ROBINSON, 2002).

Visually classified on a scale of 1 to 5 (Table 1), where a score of 1 indicates a cow that walks normally and a score of 5 indicates a cow with serious locomotor problems, determining the score is a quick assessment. Generally, scores of 2 and 3 are considered to be a subclinical presentation of lameness and scores of 4 and 5 represent animals that have the clinical problem of lameness. A locomotion score greater than 1 is not an indication of the cause of the problem, simply the degree of lameness the cow is showing (SPRECHER; HOSTETIER; KANEENE,1997).

Table 1 - Criteria used to assign a lameness score and clinical description for cattle.

Score	Description	Column	Evaluation
1	Normal	Straight	Normal posture with rectilinear back line in station and locomotion, firm steps with correct weight distribution and support.
2	Mild lameness	Straight or arched	Normal posture in station and slightly arched in locomotion, normal support.
3	Moderate lameness	Arched	Bowed posture in station and locomotion, slight change in stride.
4	Severe lameness	Arched	Arching of the body in station and locomotion, evident asymmetry of support sparing limbs, with shorter support time for injured limbs.
5	Severe lameness	Arched on 3 legs	Inability to support or bear the weight of the injured limbs, reluctance or refusal to move.

Source: adapted from Sprecher, Hostetier, and Kaneene (1997).

Table 2 shows the locomotion score with the animal standing still and moving. We can see that in score 2, when the animal is stationary, we don't notice the arching of the back when the animal is stationary, which shows that the locomotion score should also be carried out with the animal in motion.

According to Juarez and Robinson (2002), the locomotion score of individual cows can be used to select cows that need a hoof examination to assess the highest locomotion scores before they become clinically lame. In work completed on a dairy farm in California, cows that had locomotion scores of 3 were four times more likely to reach scores of 4 or 5, one month after being assessed.

Using the locomotion score as a tool, a reduction in dry matter intake (DMI) and milk production caused by lameness was observed (Figure 2). The data was collected from dairy farms in California (JUAREZ and ROBINSON, 2002).

Chart 2 - Observation of the locomotion score.

	Stop	Walking
Locomotion score 1 The line of the back remains straight in any position. All paws are planted firmly on the ground.		
Locomotion score 2 The line of the back is slightly arched when the animal walks. 0 support on the ground is not normal.		
Locomotion score 3 The line of the back is arched in any position. The stride is shorter with one paw.		
Locomotion score 4 The line of the back is always arched. Protecting the injured leg by putting less weight on it.		
Locomotion score 5 The line of the back is always arched. The animal refuses to stand on one leg.		

Source: adapted from Sprecher, Hostetier and Kaneene (1997).

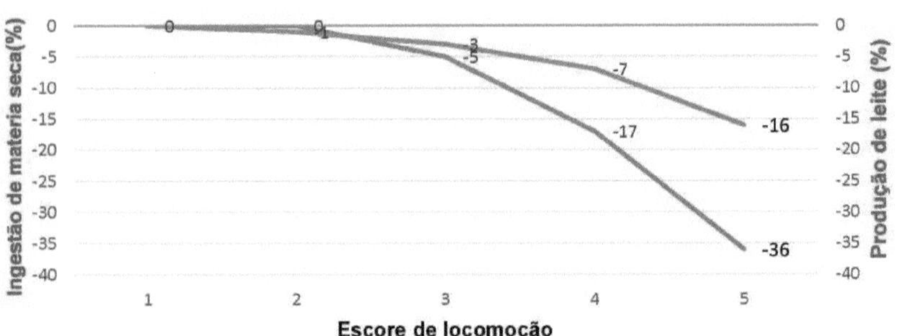

Figure 2 - Reduction in dry matter intake and milk production, related to the locomotion score.

As cows mobilise body fat and proteins to sustain milk production at higher levels, this graph does not show such a reduction in milk production, at least at the beginning of lameness, as there are still energy reserves. There is also an opposite correlation between the locomotion score and the body score, while the locomotion score increases, the body score decreases (JUAREZ and ROBINSON, 2002).

2.1.1.2Systems   for assessing the locomotion score

Most of the time, the locomotion score is carried out visually, **"manually", as it is called.** With new technologies, there are now **"automatic" locomotion scoring systems, where lameness is detected** before the animals show clinical signs. Schlageter-Tello et. al. (2014) carried out a review comparing manual and automatic locomotion scoring systems published to date, and found twenty-five manual systems in 244 articles, with the most widely used (28% of references) being the five-point system, which assesses walking asymmetry, reluctance to bear weight and arching of the spine.

Fifteen types of automatic systems were found, which can be classified into three methods: the kinetic method, which measures the force of walking; the kinematic method, which measures time and distance, associating limb movement and posture; and the indirect method, which uses production data and animal behaviour assessment as indicators of deviations in locomotion (SCHLAGETER-TELLO et. al., 2014).

Evaluating the locomotion score should be a priority task for dairy farmers. However, as the number of cows per herd is increasing, producers have less time available to carry out manual evaluation. This is one of the main reasons for the development of automatic locomotion score systems. The automatic system collects cow locomotion data using sensors. The data from these sensors is analysed using mathematical algorithms, where the system records a walking pattern and evaluates any deviations in the cows' locomotion (SCHLAGETER-TELLO, 2014).

Bicalho et al. (2007) carried out a study comparing the manual or visual locomotion score and the automatic locomotion score using the Stepmetrix system to detect painful lesions on cows' digits. The most common lesions found were sole ulcers and white line disease, respectively. Comparing the systems, they concluded that when carried out by trained professionals, the visual system is more accurate than the automatic one.

2.1.2 Stool score

Faeces are the mirror of the digestive system. Looking closely at the faeces gives us an indication of whether or not the diet is balanced, by looking at the consistency and digestion of the food that has been eaten. Consistency refers to the ratio between the amount of solid and the amount of water. If there is an abnormal breakdown of food, the intestinal contents will retain more water, making the faeces soft. Other reasons for faeces becoming soft include the presence of toxins or excess minerals in the diet (HULSEN, 2007).

The stool score is an auxiliary tool for determining how the cow's feed is being digested, whether the feed has the correct balance of nutrients (proteins, fibres and carbohydrates) and whether **water intake is adequate (TIBRU, 2010).** When assessing food digestion, look for undigested pieces of food. Ideally, every component of the diet should be digested. If some parts are not digested, either they are not digestible or there has not been enough time for complete digestion to take place. The latter occurs, for example, when the digestion rate for the energy and protein components are not in balance (feed formulation). From the moment the food is ingested, it takes one and a half to three days for it to be transformed into faeces (HULSEN, 2007).

By washing a sample of manure in a sieve you can get a good impression of how the feed is being digested and how much the cow is ruminating. Less than half of the faeces should remain in the sieve. Pieces of whole feed, such as corn kernels, that should have been digested must not be found. The fibre must show signs of having been chewed and digested. Faeces samples on the gloved hand provide similar information to the sieve (HULSEN, 2007).

2.1.2.1 Stool score classification

The faeces score is classified in two ways. One way is by looking closely at and feeling the fresh faeces with your hands to assess digestion, and the other way is by observing the consistency of the cows' fresh faeces, and you can step on the faeces with a boot for a better assessment. Both methods are graded on a five-point scale. Only fresh faeces should be analysed (ZAAIJER; NOORDHUIZEN, 2001).

2.1.2.1.1 Faeces score to assess digestion.

In score 1, the faeces are shiny, look like a creamy, homogeneous solution. There are no particles of undigested food that can be felt or seen. This is the ideal score for milking and dry cows (Figure 3).

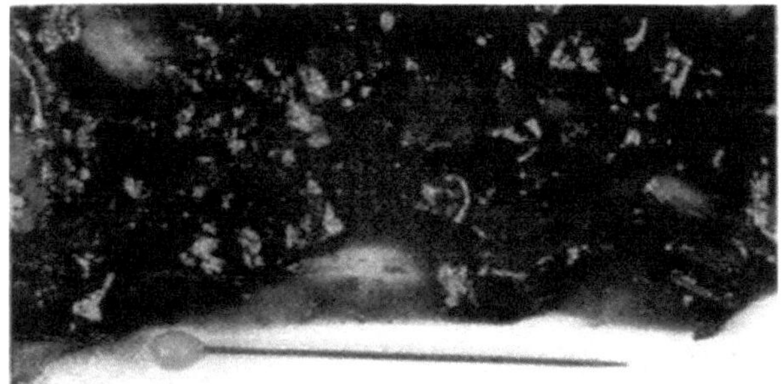

Figure 3 - Faeces score 1, assessing digestion.
Source: Adapted from Zaaijer and Noordhuizen (2001).

In score 2 the faeces are shiny and a smooth, homogeneous shape is felt. There are some undigested food particles that can be seen and felt. Still acceptable for milking and dry cows (Figure 4).

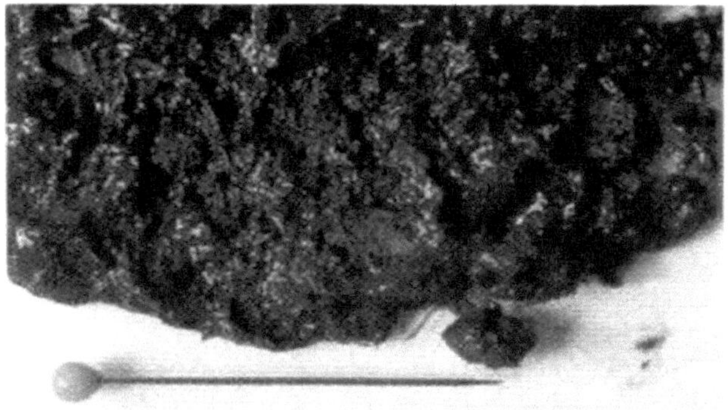

Figure 4 - Faeces score 2, assessing digestion.
Source: Adapted from Zaaijer and Noordhuizen (2001).

At score 3 the faeces appear a little more compact and inhomogeneous. After closing and opening the hand, pieces of undigested fibre remain stuck to the fingers. These faeces are acceptable for heifers and dry cows, but not for lactating cows (Figure 5).

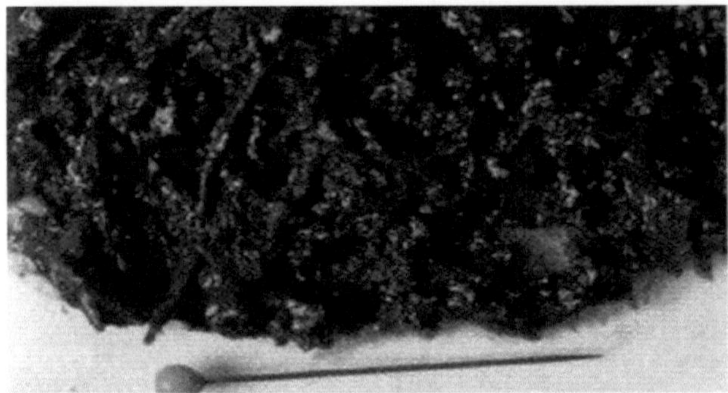

Figure 5 - Faeces score 3, assessing digestion.
Source: Adapted from Zaaijer and Noordhuizen (2001).

In score 4 the faeces are compact in appearance and contain some very coarse undigested food particles, which are clearly visible. After closing and opening the hand, a ball of undigested food remains in the hand, in which case the diet should be adjusted (Figure 6).

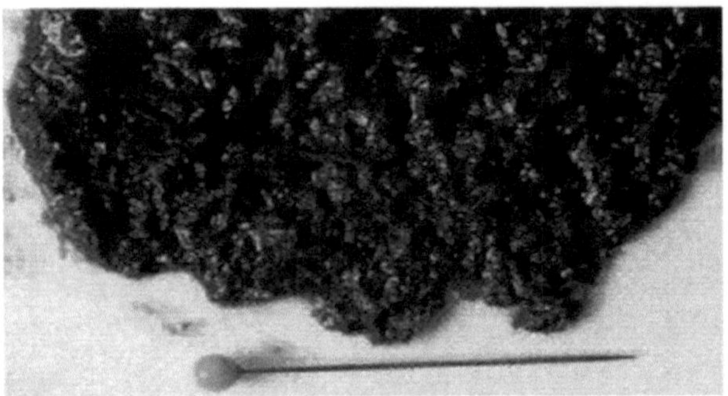

Figure 6 - Faeces score 4, assessing digestion.
Source: Adapted from Zaaijer and Noordhuizen (2001).

At score 5, coarse food particles can be felt in the faeces. Undigested dietary components are clearly visible. The faeces have a compact appearance, in which case the diet should be adjusted (Figure 7).

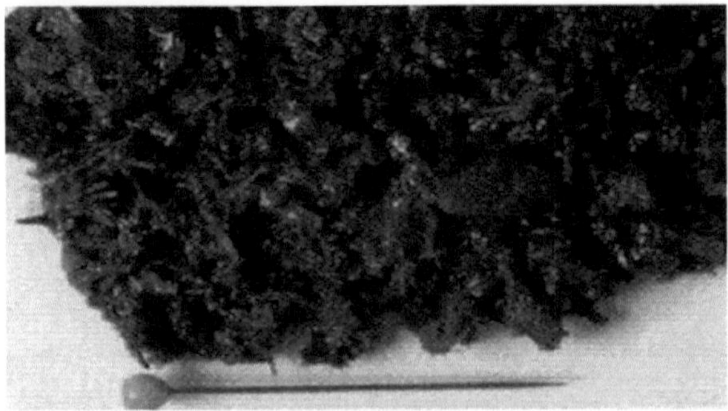

Figure 7 - Faeces score 5, assessing digestion.

2.1.2.1.2 Stool score assessing consistency.

Score 1: faeces with a very liquid consistency. When the animal is defecating, an "arc" of faeces is clearly formed on its croup. Diets with an excess of protein, starch and minerals or a lack of fibre can cause this type of stool. In general, faeces from animals with diarrhoea fit this score (Figure 8).

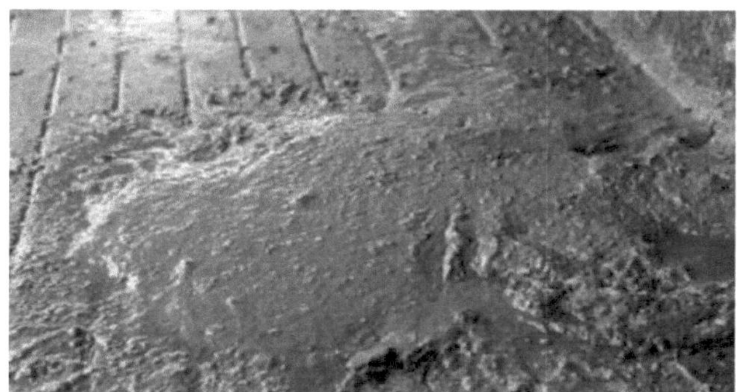

Figure 8 - Stool score 1, assessing consistency.
Source: Adapted from Zaaijer and Noordhuizen (2001).

Score 2: the faeces are still more liquid than indicated, they can run and spread when they fall on the floor. Once it has fallen to the ground, the faeces content is unlikely to form a "pile" more than 2.5 cm high. Animals on new pastures may have this score. Diets low in fibre or with little effective fibre can also cause this type of faeces (Figure 9).

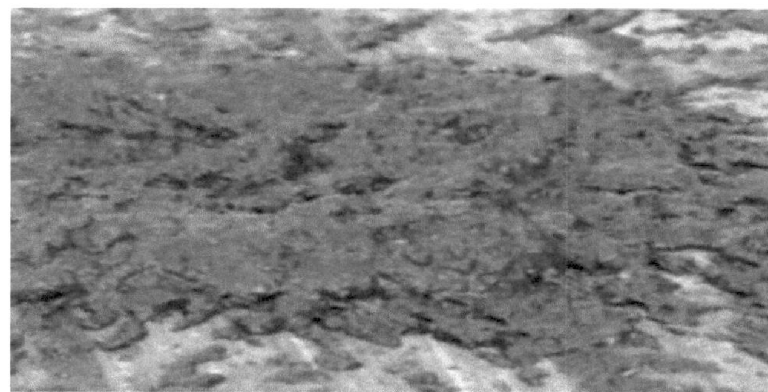

Figure 9 - Stool score 2, assessing consistency.
Source: Adapted from Zaaijer and Noordhuizen (2001).

Score 3: this is the ideal score for dairy cows. The faeces have a good consistency. When they fall to the ground, the faeces can form "piles" 4 to 5 cm high. They can have numerous concentric circles with a slight depression in the middle and unlike the previous scores, splashes of this type of faeces will stick to surfaces such as walls, gates and the boots of the professional carrying out the assessment (Figure 10).

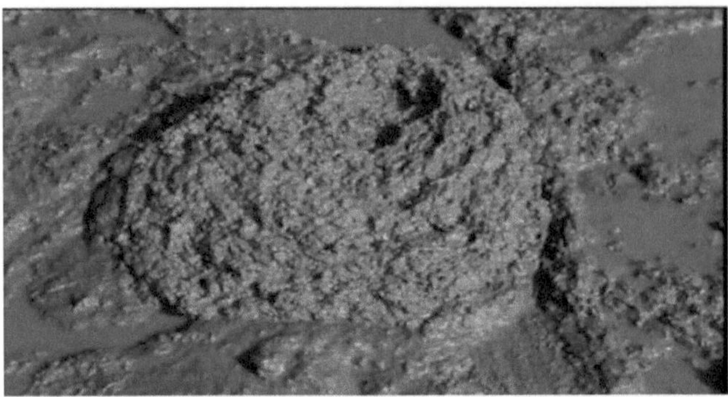
Figure 10 - Stool score 3, assessing consistency.
Source: Adapted from Zaaijer and Noordhuizen (2001).

Score 4: at this score, the faeces are already more solid and thick. The "piles" of faeces deposited on the ground reach a height of more than 5cm. Heifers and dry cows generally have this type of faeces, which indicates that they are receiving diets with lower quality forage and/or a lack of protein. Improving forage quality, increasing the amount of grain or protein can reduce this score (Figure 11).

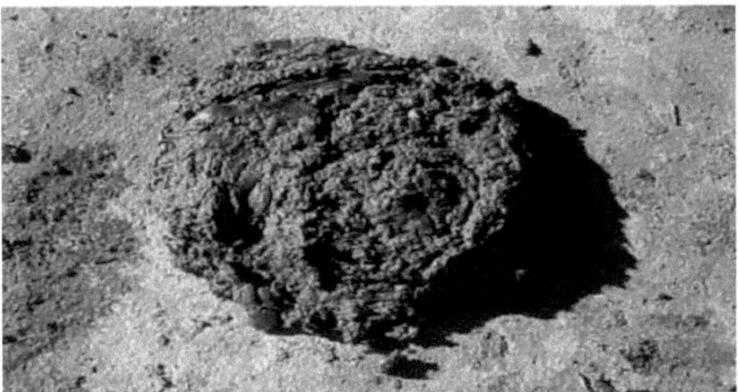
Figure 11 - Stool score 4, assessing consistency.
Source: Adapted from Zaaijer and Noordhuizen (2001).

Score 5: these faeces are already very dry, in which case dry faecal cakes are clearly formed. Animals with this type of stool may be receiving diets with very low fibre quality, such as straw or dehydrated feed, and lack of water intake. Animals with some kind of digestive blockage may also have faeces with this score (Figure 12).

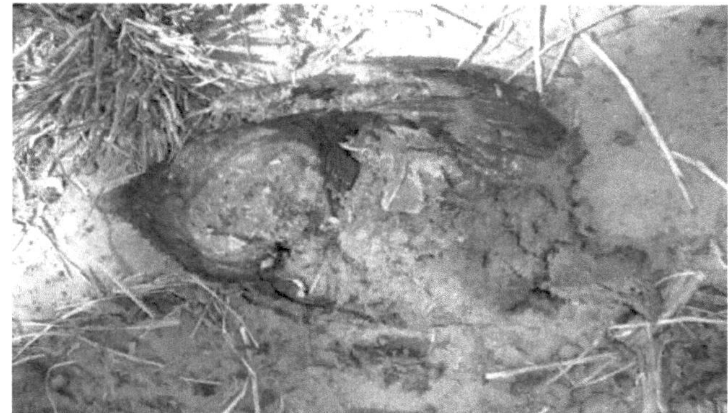

Figure 12 - Stool score 5, assessing consistency.
Source: Adapted from Zaaijer and Noordhuizen (2001).

Faecal scores of 1 and 5 are undesirable and may reflect a health problem in addition to dietary limitations. Scores below score 2 and above score 4 may indicate a need to balance the diet. Increasing the amount of degradable, soluble or total protein, decreasing the amount or physical form of fibre, increasing the level of starch, decreasing the particle size of grains (such as fine grinding or steam degradation), and over-consumption of minerals (mainly potassium and sodium) can cause a decrease in the stool score (HUTJENS, 2010).

A faeces score containing large amounts of undigested maize or with a pH below 6.0 indicates that there is an excess of grain or non-fibrous carbohydrates in the diet. It also indicates that acidosis could be a potential problem, resulting in low fat or protein content and fat inversions in the milk analysis. Stokes et al. (2000) described the indicated faeces score for each phase (Table 3).

Table 3 - Correlation at each stage with faecal score.

Phase	Score
Dry cows	3,5
Dry cows in late pregnancy	3
New mums	2,5
High-producing cows	3
Cows at the end of lactation	3,5

Source: Stokes et al.(2000).

Stallings (1993) carried out a study comparing different diets with faecal score, and found that cows fed the lactation diet were more likely to have more fluid faeces than cows fed diets with a higher fibre content; however, faecal dry matter had no relationship with faecal score.

High levels of rumen-degradable protein supplements can result in apparently more fluid faeces, probably as a result of increased water consumption in an effort to eliminate excess nitrogen through the faeces. There is a difference between cows, sometimes fed similar diets but with slightly different faecal scores. Sudden changes in faecal score can be an indicator of changes in feed composition or that the animal is ill (STALLINGS, 1993).

Faeces can also be assessed and scored based on their consistency, which can indicate imbalances in the diet and signal possible problems. Table 4 lists faecal consistency scores and descriptions as well as example situations when certain faecal consistencies can occur. Various stages of production in a cow correlate with suggested faecal scores (Stokes et al., 2000).

Table 4 - Faecal consistency scores, descriptions and examples.

Score	Description	Example
1	Thin, fluid, green	Sick cows, not eating, grazing cows
2	Loose, with ripples, no definition of shape	Newly calved cows, grazing cows
3	Piles 2.5 to 4 cm high, undulating, 2 to 4 concentric rings	Recommended for high production cows
4	5 to 7.5 cm pile	Dry cow, low in protein and high in fibre
5	Larger 7.5 cm battery	High forage diets, sick cows

Source: Stokes et al. (2000).

2.1.2.2 Faeces colouring

The colour of faeces is influenced by the feed, the amount of bile, and the rate of passage. Faeces from grazing cows are dark green, while hay-based diets are brown. Grain-based diets are more grey. Slower passage rates darken the faeces and they become ball-shaped with a greyish colour.

shine on the surface due to the mucus coating. Score 1 may be lighter in colour due to more water and less bile content. Bleeding in the small intestine causes black and dark stools, while bleeding in the rectum results in a brownish-red colour or reddish streaks (HUTJENS, 2010).

2.1.3 Body condition score

The body condition score (BCS) can be a good management tool, where it is used to monitor the amount and mobilisation of adipose tissue in the body and therefore indicates the negative energy balance (NEB) of cows in early lactation (LAWLOR, 2004). Edmondson et al. (1989), reported that ECC is a subjective method of assessing the amount of metabolisable energy stored in adipose tissue and muscle (body reserves) in a live animal.

This condition score method is based on a visual and tactile assessment of body fat reserves in the back and pelvic region and the ECC is usually scored on a scale of 1 to 5 points

(WILDMAN et. al., 1982).

According to Hulsen (2007), the body condition score provides a subjective estimate of the amount of fat between the ischiums and the base of the tail, over the hip area, and covering the lumbar vertebrae (Chart 5).

Changes in body condition take place over weeks or months. The condition score increases when a cow's energy intake is too high and decreases when its intake is too low. A lean cow has a score of 1, an obese cow has a score of 5. In this way, a standard classification has been developed that makes it possible to follow trends in body condition and to feed cows according to their energy needs (HULSEN, 2007).

Cows that are overweight at the time of calving will decrease their dry matter intake post-calving. Thin cows also have lower immunity, reducing their resistance to disease. Along with this come problems with fertility, which include cystic ovaries, inactive ovaries, little or no oestrus and a poor quality corpus luteum. The condition score should not decrease by more than 0.75 points over the course of a lactation (HULSEN, 2007).

Chart 5 - Body condition score in dairy cows.

Score	Condition	Description	Visual
1	Slim	Base of tail - deep cavity without subcutaneous fatty tissue. Very subtle skin, often with rough fur. Loin - prominent spine and pronounced horizontal process.	
2	Moderate	Base of tail - shallow cavity but prominent ischia; a little subcutaneous fatty tissue. Soft skin. Loin - Horizontal processes can be identified individually with rounded ends.	
3	Good	Base of tail - layer of fatty tissue along the entire area and smooth skin. Loin - the end of the horizontal process can only be felt with pressure; only a slight depression in the loin.	

| 4 | Fat | Base of tail - completely full and folds and parts with obvious fatty tissue.

Loin - can't feel the processes and will have a completely rounded appearance. | |
| 5 | Obese | Base of tail - buried in fatty tissue, pelvis impalpable, even with firm pressure. | |

Source: Hulsen (2007).

The body condition score has gained greater acceptance as a tool for evaluating energy balance, body composition and body reserves instead of live weight in dairy cows. Lactating cows use tissue reserves to support milk production, so the BCS can serve as a useful measure of tissue mobilisation (OTTO, 1990).

Edmondson et al (1989) developed a system of drawings to classify the body condition score, using scores from 1 to 5, as shown in Figure 13.

The body condition score system is a means of accurately determining the body condition of dairy cows, regardless of **the animal's** body weight and **size. Olechnowicz and Jaskowski** (2014) found a significant relationship between body condition score and lameness, where cows that had some degree of lameness had a lower body condition score compared to healthy cows. Ferreira et al (2013) assessed the impact of body condition on the pregnancy rate of Nelore cows, and found a statistical difference, **where cows with a score < 2.5 > 2.0 had a** lower **pregnancy rate** compared to **cows with a score of 3.0.**

Nutrition plays a fundamental role in regulating reproductive processes. The effects of nutrition are measurable through cow characteristics such as ECC. A decline in ECC of more than 0.5 points is known to have negative effects on fertility. It is therefore used as a decision-making tool in feeding management. However, changes in ECC take weeks or months, which is too long for precise and timely adjustments in feed management (ZAAIJER; NOORDHUIZEN, 2001). A body condition score is equal to 45 to 65kg of gain in body weight. Larger-framed cows need more additional body weight to increase a point, compared to smaller-framed or narrow cows (KELLOGG, 2010).

A properly nourished herd avoids extremes in body condition score, i.e. 2 or less, and above 4. Therefore, the feeding programme should be adjusted so that the diets are balanced according to their level of production. Older cows should calve with a BCC of around 3.5. However, fat cows should be avoided at calving, as they are more prone to metabolic problems such as dystocia or calving-related problems, retained placenta, hypocalcaemia, ketosis and fallen cow syndrome. Table 6 shows the ideal score for each stage of the cow.

Table 6 - Ideal body condition score

Stage of lactation	Score
Drying	3,5
Childbirth	3,5
One month after giving birth	2,5-3,0
Average lactation	3,0
Late lactation	3,25 - 3,75

Source: Kellogg (2010).

Figure 14 shows the typical curve for a lactating cow and the energy consumption and body weight for the cow. Feeding a high-producing cow requires more energy than a lower-producing cow. She may not be able to consume enough to meet her energy needs and so mobilise from reserves.

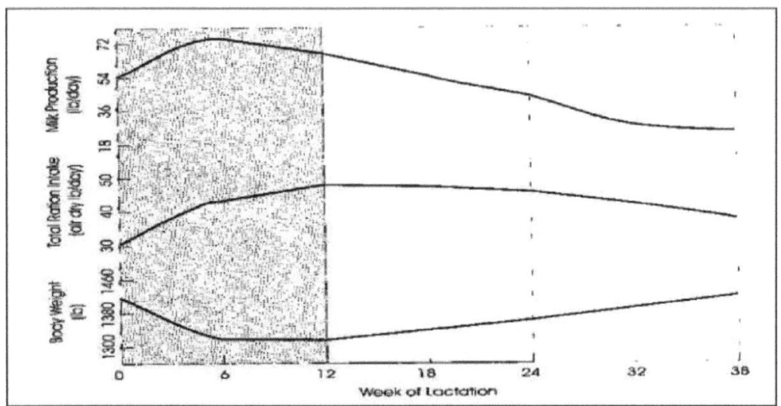

Figure 14 - Effect of stage of lactation on milk production, feed intake and body condition.

Source: Kellogg (2010).

2.1.4 Trough score

Many variables can affect feed intake, including animal factors, climate, feed ingredients and characteristics, water supply, feeding trough design and feeding management systems. Proper trough management depends on the person responsible for feeding the animals understanding how these variables affect DM intake and recognising problems that occur. Dry matter intake is mainly affected by milk production (45% variation), feed and feed management (22% variation), body weight (17% variation), climate (10% variation), and body condition score (6% variation) (ROSELER et al., 1997).

The trough score is used to maximise feed consumption and minimise waste and spoilage of the diet provided. Evaluating the trough score automatically analyses the content of leftovers and the quality of the feed that has been offered. According to Bierman (2001), the trough score is the supervision and execution to determine, in an acceptable and coherent way, the amount of food that an animal can consume in a given period of time. The management of the trough represents a great challenge, as the person carrying it out must have a good understanding of the concept, so as not to jeopardise the cows' diet.

The University of South Dakota has developed a specific trough score system where five points are used (Table 7). By providing a detailed description of the leftovers from the trough, this system reduces the variability of feed supply, which is good for the animals. These records are used for each feeding of the diet and at least four days of records should be analysed to determine a feed change. Keeping these trough score records every day will help determine feed conversions (in the case of beef cattle), seasonal variability, production costs, as well as assessing how often feed needs to be provided (BOLSEN; POLLARD, 2004).

Table 7 - Trough score, University of South Dakota.

0	No feed left in the trough
1	Scattered food (less than 5% of the amount supplied)
2	Thin layer (< 5 cm) remaining (5-10% of the amount supplied)
3	Medium layer (between 5-8 cm) remaining (around 25% of the amount supplied)
4	Thick layer (> 8 cm) remaining (about 50% of the amount supplied)
5	Intact food

Source: adapted from Bolsen and Pollard (2004).

Trough scores of 0 and 1 indicate that the herd is undernourished. If the cows are consuming the last 5 per cent of the amount of feed provided, it means that they are not eating to their full potential, as this is a sign of poorly palatable, spoilt or inferior quality forage. Another important management action is to move the feed in the trough at least 3-4 times a day, usually before the animals come back from milking. This procedure stimulates the animals' consumption of food. Any leftovers from the diets of lactating cows should be removed daily before the start of the next day's treatment and can be used as part of the diet of growing heifers (BOLSEN; POLLARD, 2004).

Researchers at Ohio State University (USA) have also described a way of evaluating trough management. For it to be implemented successfully, the keeper must have complete control over the management and supply of the diet. Firstly, the level of leftovers must be regularised at between 2% and 3% per tract and the diet must be fractioned as many times as possible within the farm's routine. Table 8 shows the scores according to the Ohio State University researchers.

Chart 8 - Trough management, Ohio State University.

Score	Description of the trough	Action
0	Empty trough for more than 1 hour (between treatments)	Increase the quantity supplied by between 1% and 2%
1	Empty trough for less than 1 hour (between treatments)	Maintain the quantity supplied
2	Presence of small feed particles in the trough (less than 2.5 cm of feed layer in the trough)	Maintain quantity supplied
3	More than a 2.5 cm layer of food in the trough	Decrease the amount supplied in 1 % a 2%

Source: http://www.milkpoint.com.br/radar-tecnico/nutricao/novos-conceitos-bordando-o- monitoring-the-diet-echo-echo-echo-echo-part-2-18602n.aspx

Bierman and Pritchard (1996) used a trough management strategy where one group of beef cattle had ad libitum access to feed and another group had a clean trough management strategy (troughs were clean for 70% of the 24-hour period). The cattle fed with the clean trough management strategy had a 10% reduction in IMS, and an 11% improvement in feed efficiency resulting in 24.60 dollars more per head compared to the ad libitum group (Figure 15).

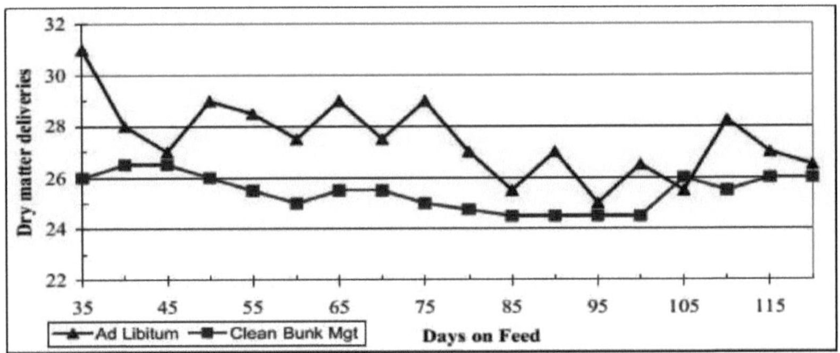

Figure 15 - Trough management strategy compared to ad libitum.
Source: Bierman and Pritchard (1996).

The trough score is not only used to observe the amount of food in the trough, but also to know whether quality, nutritious, fresh, consistent food is being provided in a way that maximises consumption and minimises waste and spoilage (LOY, 1997).

1.1.5 Rumen score

The rumen score is an indication of feed intake and the rate of feed passage over the last few hours. The rumen score is assessed from the cow's left flank (paralumbar fossa) and requires observation from the animal's left side. What will be observed is rumen filling. Rumen filling is based on a combination of the amount of feed consumed, the speed of digestion, and the rate at which the feed passes into the abomasum and intestine. The rate of digestion and the rate of passage are affected by the characteristics of the components of the diet (fast or slow fermenting feeds), the particle size, and the balance between the different components of the feed in the rumen (HULSEN, 2007).

Burfeind et al. (2010), in an experiment comparing dry matter intake with rumen score, found that observing rumen fill score is a reasonable estimate of IMS, as significant differences in measurements of the paralumbar fossa were observed in a short space of time. Furthermore, in order to determine the rumen score, the cow must not be contracting the rumen, as this could lead to errors in visualisation. They therefore recommend that the score is always taken at the same time of day.

1.1.5.1 Rumen score classification

According to Zaaijer and Noordhuizenv (2001), the rumen score is classified by looking at the paralumbar fossa between the last rib, the transverse processes and the iliac bone. They are classified as follows:

Score 1: the paralumbar fossa is visualised as very empty; the paralumbar fossa has a cavity more than a palm's width behind the last rib and also the width of a hand inside and under the transverse processes. The fossa looks like a rectangle when viewed from the left side of the cow. These cows usually eat little or not at all due to illness (Figure 16).

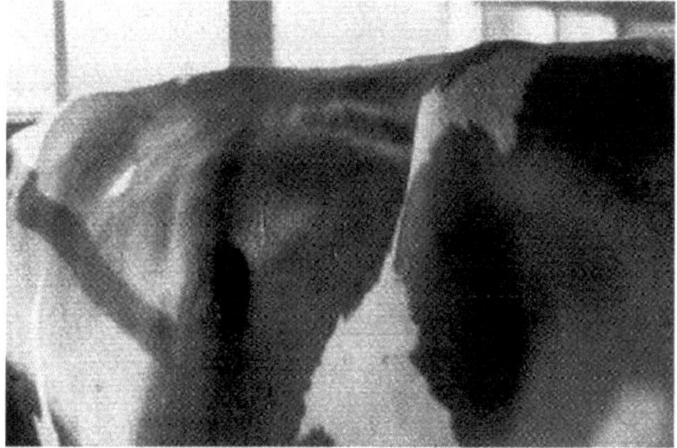

Figure 16 - Rumen score 1.
Source: Adapted from Zaaijer and Noordhuizenv (2001).

Score 2: Paralumbar fossa with a cavity the width of a hand behind the last rib and, to a lesser extent, inwards under the transverse processes. Standing on the left side of the cow, this area looks like a triangle. This condition is often observed in normal cows in the first week postpartum. When rumen fill does not increase after this period, it is an indication of low feed intake (Figure 17).

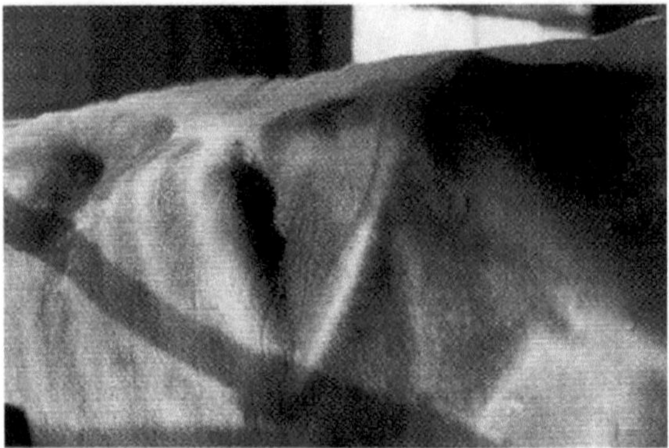

Figure 17 - Rumen score 2.
Source: Adapted from Zaaijer and Noordhuizenv (2001).

Score 3: the paralumbar fossa has a cavity smaller than the width of a hand behind the last rib and falls about the width of a hand vertically downwards from the transverse processes and protrudes outwards. This is the desired rumen fill for lactating cows with adequate dry matter intake (Figure 18).

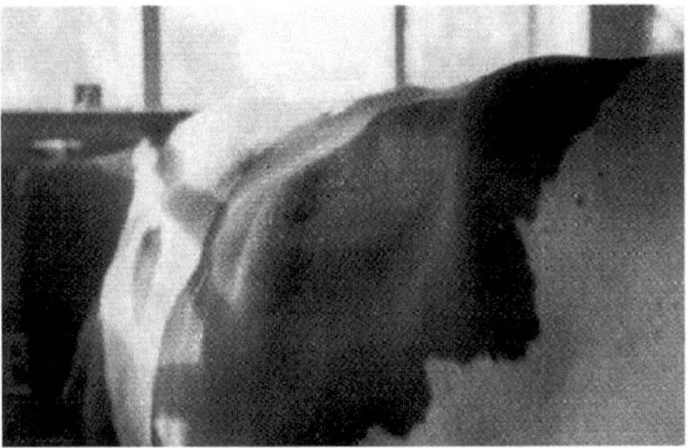

Figure 18 - Rumen score 3.
Source: Adapted from Zaaijer and Noordhuizenv (2001).

Score 4: the skin covers the paralumbar fossa, the area behind the last rib and the transverse processes, due to a distended rumen. Dry cows and cows in late lactation should show this score (Figure 19).

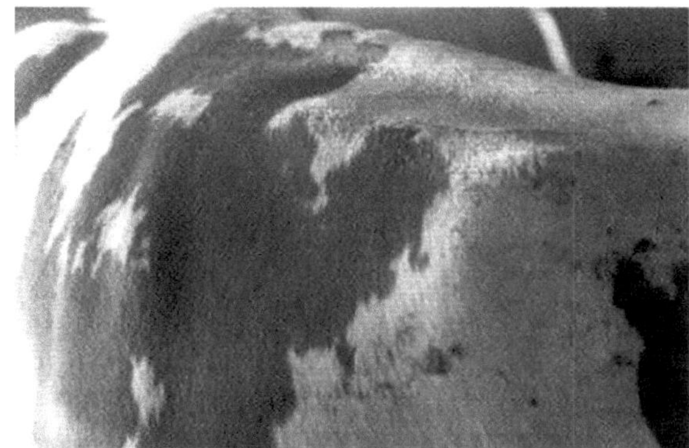

Figure 19 - Rumen score 4.
Source: Adapted from Zaaijer and Noordhuizenv (2001).

Score 5: rumen is very distended and almost obliterates the fossa; the last rib and the transverse processes are not visible. This is the score for dry cows (Figure 20).

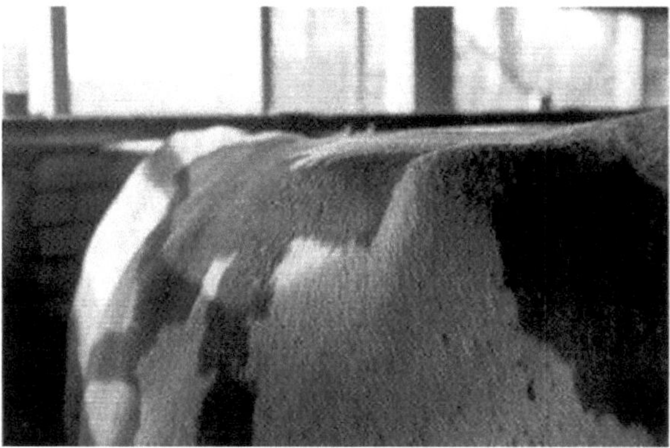

Figure 20 - Rumen score 5.
Source: Adapted from Zaaijer and Noordhuizenv (2001).

CHAPTER 3

PRESENTATION OF THE FIELD ORGANISATION

3.1 FIELD ORGANISATION IDENTIFICATION DATA

3.1.1 Company name

Company name: NUTRE SAÚDE E PRODUÇÃO ANIMAL

Address: Rua Adelarte de Bortoli, n. 601

Postcode: 85,575-000 - São Jorge D' Oeste-PR

Phone: (46) 3534-1728

E-mail: nutresaojorge@gmail.com

3.1.2 Internship supervisor

Abílio Galvão Trindade Ferreira, CRMV - 3951 - PR Marcelo Trindade Ferreira, CRMV - 6635 - PR

3.2 PRESENTATION OF THE FIELD ORGANISATION

NUTRE Saúde e Produção Animal is based in the municipality of **São Jorge D'Oeste (PR). It was founded on 4 April 2003 and offers services** related to technical assistance on dairy and beef cattle farms, covering the areas of production, reproduction, nutrition, preventive veterinary medicine, clinic, surgery and rural management. It provides assistance to properties in the municipalities of São Jorge do Oeste, Francisco Beltrão, São João, Salto do Lontra, Nova Esperança do Sudoeste, Dois Vizinhos, Verê, Sulina and Coronel Vivida. It currently has five veterinarians, three of whom live **in São Jorge do Oeste, one in Salto do Lontra** and one in Francisco Beltrão, and a **zootechnician who lives in São Jorge do Oeste.**

The company NUTRE Saúde e Produção Animal, with headquarters in Rua Adelarte de **Bortoli, in the municipality of São Jorge D' Oeste, is overseen by the following doctors**

Veterinarians Abílio Galvão Trindade Ferreira and Marcelo Trindade Ferreira. São Jorge

D'oeste is a municipality located in the south-western region of Paraná, also **known as the "Land of the Iguaçu Lakes". It has an area of 379.546** km^2 with a population of approximately 9,000 inhabitants. The economy is based on agriculture and livestock, with a large number of cattle.

Approximately 40,000 head of cattle, around 10,000 of which are dairy cattle.

CHAPTER 4

DEVELOPMENT OF THE SUPERVISED CURRICULAR INTERNSHIP

4.1   PRESENTATION OF THE ACTIVITIES CARRIED OUT

The supervised curricular internship was carried out at the NUTRE-PR company from 2 March to 2 May 2015, totalling 61 days with a workload of 40 hours a week, giving a total of 360 hours of supervised curricular internship. The activities carried out are summarised in the following tables:

Table 1 - List of activities carried out and/or monitored during the supervised curricular internship in Veterinary Medicine at the NUTRE company, from 2nd March to 2nd May 2015

Activities	Number	%
Reproductive Clinic	939	47,74
Medical Clinic	215	10,93
Surgical Clinic	16	0,81
Preventive Medicine	797	40,52
Total	**1967**	**100**

Source: Tomasini (2015).

Table 2 - List of surgical activities carried out and/or monitored during the supervised curricular internship in Veterinary Medicine at NUTRE, from 2nd March to 2nd May 2015.

Activities	Number	%
Orchiectomy	5	31,25
Displacement of the abomasum	6	37,50
Digit amputation	1	6,25
Removal of a supernumerary roof	1	6,25
Removal of a 3^a eyelid tumour	2	12,50
Persistent urachus	1	6,25
Total	**16**	**100**

Source: Tomasini (2015).

Table 3 - List of activities in the area of reproductive clinic carried out and/or monitored during the supervised curricular internship in Veterinary Medicine at the NUTRE company, from 2nd March to 2nd May 2015.

Activities	Number	%
Abortion	3	0,32
Childbirth assistance	13	1,38
Pregnancy Diagnosis	238	25,35
Pregnancy Diagnosis with Ultrasound	54	5,75
Andrological examination	70	7,45
Gynaecological examination	475	50,59

	14	1,49
Puerperal endometritis	14	1,49
IATF	52	5,54
Foetal mummification	2	0,21
Vagina/cervix prolapse	1	0,11
Retained placenta	17	1,81
Total	**939**	**100**

Source: Tomasini (2015).

Table 4 - List of activities in the area of preventive medicine carried out and/or monitored during the supervised curricular internship in Veterinary Medicine at the NUTRE company, from 2nd March to 2nd May 2015.

Activities	**Number**	**%**
Brucellosis tests	266	33,38
Tuberculosis tests	332	41,66
Vaccination against brucellosis	23	2,89
Vaccination against IBR, BVD and PI3	176	22,08
Total	**797**	**100**

Source: Tomasini (2015).

Table 5 - List of activities in the area of clinical medicine carried out and/or monitored during the supervised curricular internship in Veterinary Medicine at the NUTRE company, from 2nd March to 2nd May 2015.

Activities	**Number**	**%**
Actinobacillosis	2	0,93
Foot disorders	24	11,16
Artogripose	1	0,47
Non-surgical dehorning	14	6,51
Non-specific diarrhoea	2	0,93
Hypocalcaemia	9	4,19
Simple indigestion	2	0,93
Hovenia dulcis poisoning	2	0,93
Lechiguana	2	0,93
Obturator nerve injury	2	0,93
Non-specific mastitis	37	17,21
Subclinical mastitis	8	3,72
Necropsy	6	2,79
Non-specific pneumonia	59	27,44
Bovine parasitic disease	43	20,00
Keratoconjunctivitis	2	0,93
Total	**215**	**100**

Source: Tomasini (2015).

4.2   DISCUSSION OF ACTIVITIES

The scores are a means of diagnosing the farm, and are used to monitor the cows during lactation and also when they are dry. By looking at the locomotion score, we can identify which cows need clinical or preventive hoof trimming. The body condition score helps us realise which cows are too thin and which are overweight. Trough and rumen scores indicate whether the animals have been fed properly or not, and the faeces score is a reflection of how their digestion is going and whether anything is missing from the diet. Often the scores can be related, which is a good way to diagnose problems that are happening on the farm.

4.2.1 Locomotion score and trough score

Juarez et al. (2003) found lameness to be the third most important economic loss related to animal health in dairy cattle, after fertility and mastitis. Naibo (2014) also reported that locomotor problems are in third place for discarding dairy cows, after mammary gland problems and reproduction. So in addition to animal welfare, there is a great deal of economic importance involved in the animal's locomotor system.

On the farms we visited, the animals' gait was often assessed by the farmer himself, who would tell us which animal was limping, but the farmer would only diagnose when the score was 3 or 4. On the day of the technical assistance, it was always analysed whether any cows had grown hooves or were limping to some degree, requiring hoof trimming. When there were only a few animals (one or two), hoof trimming was carried out without the use of a hoof trimmer, but when there were more cases, it was carried out by a veterinarian who worked exclusively with hoof trimming, using a hydraulic hoof trimmer. During the internship, a case occurred on a property assisted by the company, where the problem of fat/protein inversion was occurring (Figure 21) and some cows appeared with grade 3 and 4 lameness. The trough score on the day the property was visited was "0", indicating that the animals were lacking feed (Figure 22).

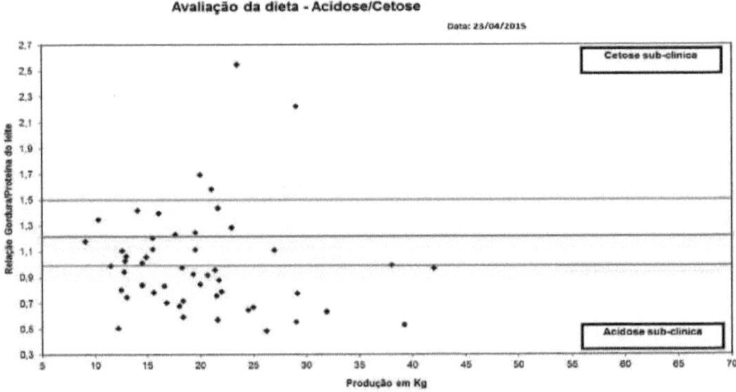

Figure 21 - Milk control, showing which cows are in acidosis or ketosis through the ratio of fat to protein. Source: Tomasini (2015).

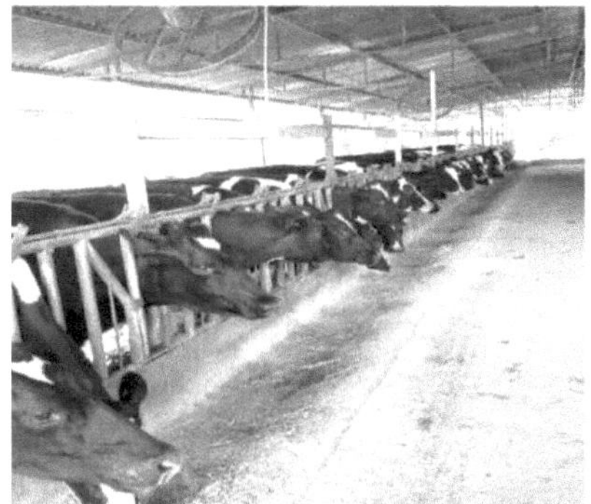

Figure 22 - Trough score "0". Trough without food "licked".

Source: Tomasini (2015).

Fat values that are 0.4 percentage **points** lower than total protein values **can be considered "inversions"** (for example, a fat content of less than 2.8 per cent associated with a total protein content of 3.2 per cent). If the protein data is expressed as true protein (not including non-protein nitrogen), fat values 0.2 percentage points lower than true protein values **are considered "inversions"**. Up to 10 per cent of lactating cows with these types of inversions are considered normal (GONZÁLEZ; DURR; FONTANELI, 2001).

The drop in fat content and/or inversions in the fat and protein content of milk are generally related to rumen acidosis and this fat depression

in milk can be explained by the theory of biohydrogenation. According to Hussein et al. (2013), when the rumen environment is modified, in diets with low fibre or poor fibre effectiveness for example, there is a change in the biohydrogenation of unsaturated fatty acids, causing the synthesis of CLA (conjugated linoleic acid) to occur, this fatty acid inhibits fat synthesis by the mammary gland. Among the alterations is the appearance of hoof problems, which is caused by rumen acidosis, where vasoactive substances (histamine and endotoxins) are released during the decline in rumen pH, as a result of bacteriolysis and tissue degradation. These substances cause vasoconstriction and dilation, which ultimately destroys the microvasculature of the chorion and causes hoof problems (BRENT, 1976).

Problems with lameness were occurring on this property, and nine animals in total were hoof trimmed. The most common lesions were white line disease and sole ulcers (Figure 23). According to Greenough (2007), vasoactive substances and endotoxins originating in the rumen as a result of acidosis, metabolic disturbances, or inflammatory processes, directly interfere with the microcirculation of the hoof or trigger the release of cytokines, which in turn affect the integrity of the hoof tissue. The result is a dysfunction or even interruption in the production of horny tissue for short or long periods and with varying degrees of severity, which results in a softening of the hoof and the appearance of diseases such as sole ulcers and white line disease.

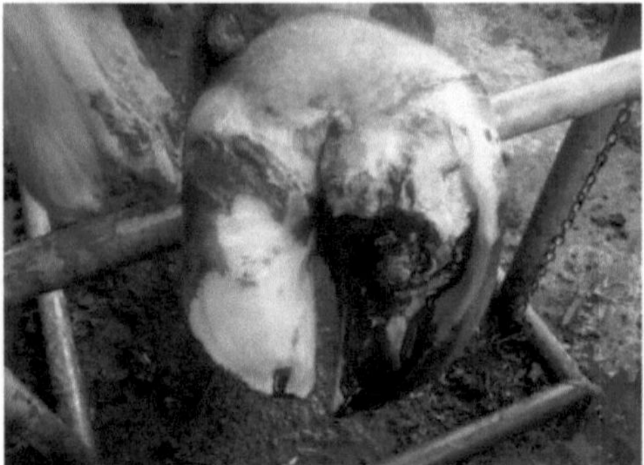

Figure 23 - Bovine hoof with sole ulcer lesion.
Source: Tomasini (2015).

Around a fortnight before the milk check, the diet was adjusted and hay was added to the total diet (Figure 24), with the aim of improving the fat/protein ratio in the milk and getting the cows out of acidosis.

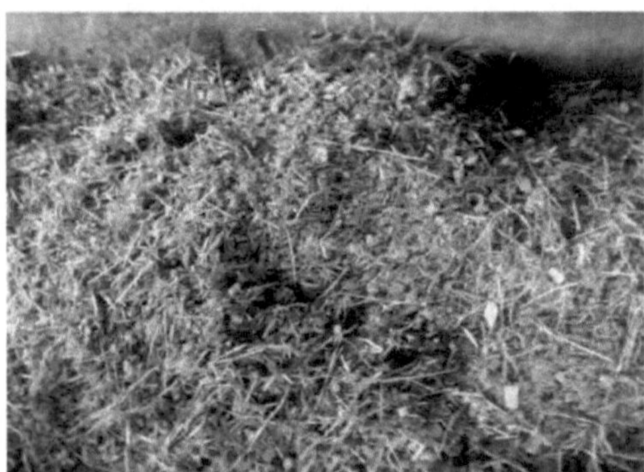

Figure 24 - Addition of hay to the total diet.
Source: Tomasini (2015).

However, as shown in the milk control in Figure 21, the cows continued to have an inversion of fat and protein, indicating acidosis. Knowing this information, a check was made to find out where the error lay. In theory, everything was fine, the diet was balanced, the feed was given three times **a day, but the trough score of "0" was not as expected. Then,** talking to the employee in charge of feeding, it was discovered that the cows were receiving the wrong amount of maize silage: on the paper it said 30kg/animal/day and what was being fed was 12kg per animal per day. In this case, as well as the lack of dry matter for the animals, the bulk/concentrate ratio was unbalanced, as the amount of concentrate in the diet was not altered, but the bulk was reduced, leaving the animals in a state of ruminal acidosis. Table 6 shows the effect of the volume/concentrate ratio on rumen fermentation, which is closely related to the case described. When there is an excess of concentrate, the fat content drops excessively, below 2.8 per cent, as well as reducing feed intake and milk production (MUHLBACH, 2000).

Table 6 - Effect of the volume:concentrate ratio on rumen fermentation.

---------------------- % of MS -------------				Chewing	pH	-------Molar %---------		Relationship
Voluminous	Concentrate	NDF	FDA	(min/day)	Rumen	Acetic	Propionic	Molar
100	0	65	41	960	7,0a	70	18	3,9
80	20	55	34	940	6,6a	67	20	3,4
60	40	45	27	900	6,2a	64	22	2,9
40	60	34	20	820	5,8	58	28	2,1b
20	80	24	13	660	5,4	48	34	1,4b
0	100	14	6	340	5,0	36	45	0,8b

a - pH range suitable for cellulose fermentation. b - molar ratio that causes a drop in milk fat %.
Adapted from Bachman (1992), in Muhlbach et al., 2000.

4.2.2 Assessment of the faeces score

On the day of the technical assistance, all the properties had their animals' faeces evaluated, so that they could get an idea of how their digestion and diet were going. According to Tibru (2010), the faeces score is an auxiliary tool for determining how the cow's food is being digested, whether the feed has the correct balance of nutrients (proteins, fibres and carbohydrates) and whether water intake is adequate.

The faeces were evaluated according to Zaaijer and Noordhuizen (2001). Depending on how the faeces score was, recommendations were made to the farmer about feeding the animals. Faecal score 1 was found in animals suffering from diarrhoea (Figure 25), in which case treatment with antibiotics was carried out. In both cases of diarrhoea, the cows were feeding on silage that was in the process of fermentation. The cows had a fever, loss of appetite and reduced milk production. Treatment was carried out with sulfa + trimethoprim in two doses of 20mg/kg at 48-hour intervals and they were also instructed to stop feeding silage. A score of 1 can also occur due to an excess of concentrate and/or a lack of fibre in the diet.

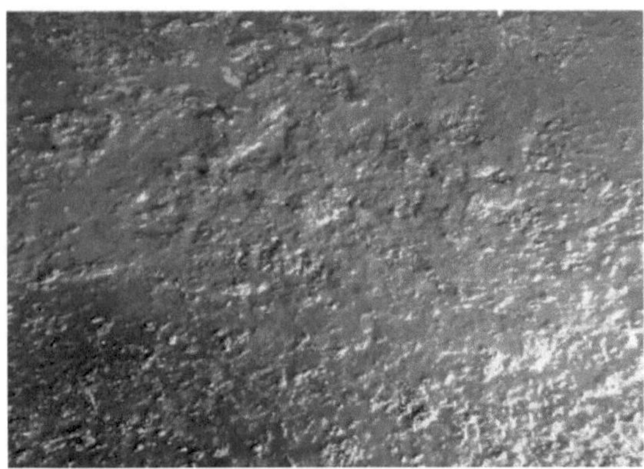
Figure 25 - Faeces score 1.
Source: Tomasini (2015)

When most of the animals had a score of around 2 (Figure 26), the particle size of the diet was assessed. If the roughage was too finely chopped, hay or soya hulls were added, with the aim of improving rumination and, consequently, digestion in these animals, which was reflected in the faeces score. According to Garleb et. al. (1998), due to its low lignin content and high proportion of digestible fibre, soybean hulls can be used as a substitute for roughage when necessary. However, this faeces score is accepted in cows in the first stage of lactation, where the diet is challenging for the cow and contains a large amount of concentrate. We can also observe this score when cows are grazing grasses at an early vegetative stage.

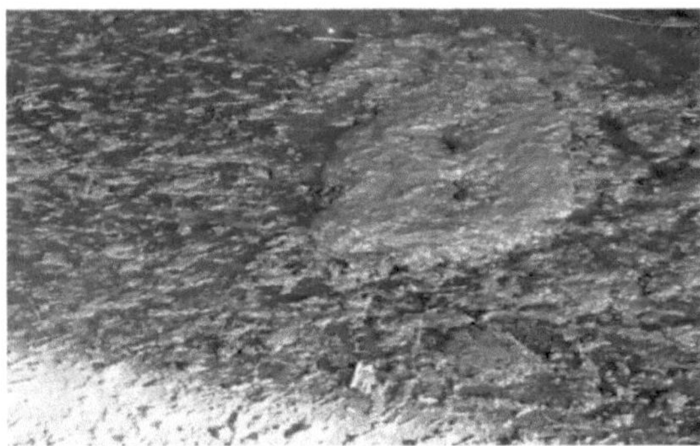
Figure 26 - Faeces score 2.
Source: Tomasini (2015).

Faeces score 3, which is ideal, was found on farms that had a balanced diet and the farmer had not made any changes without guidance (Figure 27).

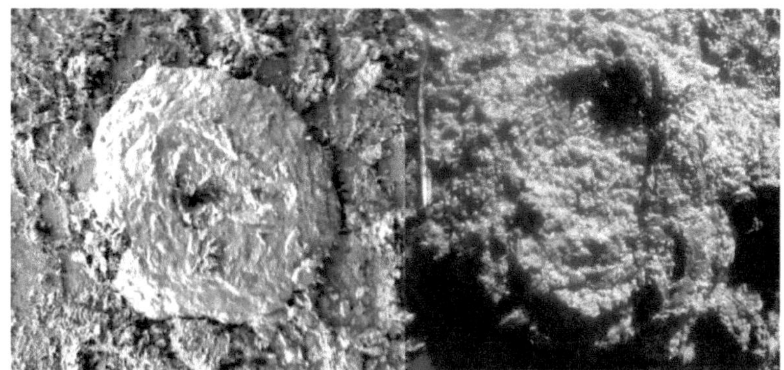
Figure 27 - Faeces score 3.
Source: Tomasini (2015).

Score 4 was generally observed in dry cows and heifers (Figure 28), as the diet of these animals does not contain a large amount of concentrate and is basically composed of fibre, in agreement with Zaaijer and Noordhuizen (2001).

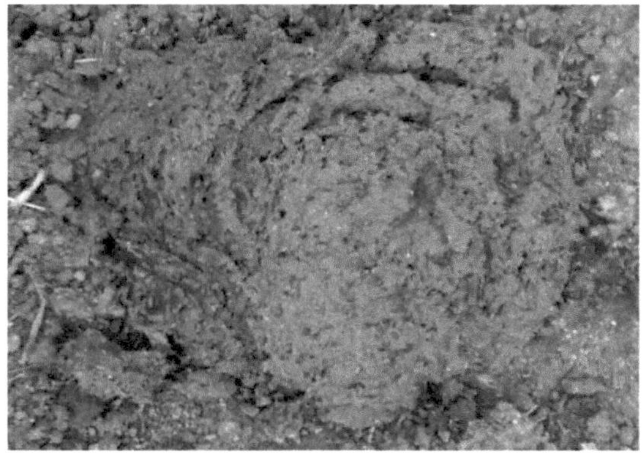
Figure 28 - Faeces score 4.
Source: Tomasini (2015).

Rarely was a score of 5 found, usually these were animals that were on low quality pasture or fibre and not fed concentrates (Figure

29). This score can be found when animals have a gastrointestinal disorder in which peristalsis is reduced, diseases with fever and spinal cord injuries that affect the digestive system can also trigger a faeces score of 5.

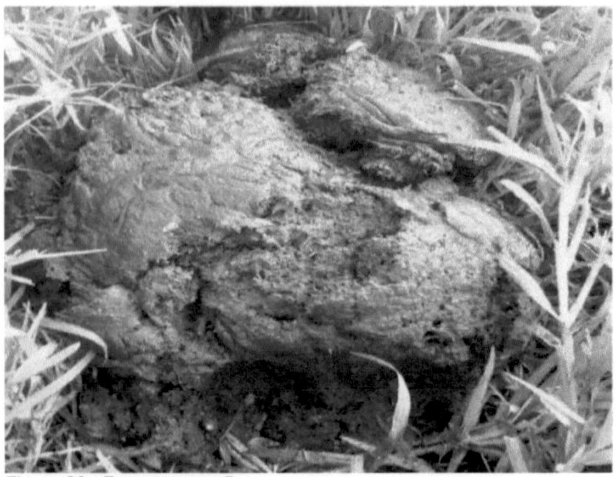
Figure 29 - Faeces score 5.
Source: Tomasini (2015).

1.1.1.1 Particle size

One of the key points for good digestive functioning in ruminants is the particle size of the diet. According to Stokes et al. (2000), the right particle size in the diet is necessary to avoid digestive problems and the production of low-fat milk. Cows require fibre and forage to stimulate chewing and saliva production, both of which are necessary for maintaining pH and rumen health.

To determine the size and quantity of particles in roughage or the total diet, Lammers, Buckmaster and Heinrichs (1996) developed the Penn State Sieve (Figure 30). The sieve consists of a series of stacked screens that separate a feed sample into various particle sizes, providing a visual, quantitative assessment of particle size distribution.

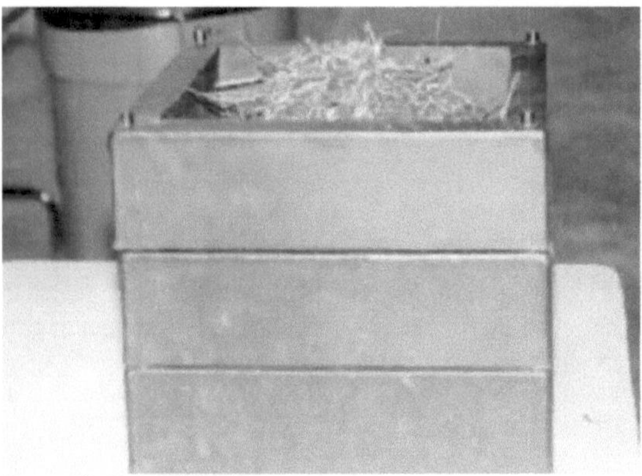
Figure 30 - Penn State sieve.
Source: Stokes et al. (2000)

The sieve separates the particles into three groups: particles larger than 19mm, between 8 and 19mm and smaller than 8mm. At the top are the particles that will form part of the "rumen mat" (a layer of long particles that floats on top of the rumen content and stimulates chewing, saliva production and rumination). The middle part identifies the portion of the diet that is moderately digestible. The last part collects particles that are easily digestible or quickly removed from the rumen (STOKES et al., 2000).

On the farms visited, when necessary, the total diet or silage was evaluated using a sieve. According to Heinrichs and Kononoff (2002), if maize silage is the only forage, at least 8% of the particles should remain in the top sieve, and at least 3% when maize silage is not the only forage. Around 45 to 65 per cent of the silage should remain in the middle sieve and 30 to 40 per cent in the lower sieve of the separator. For the total diet, the values change slightly, with 8% or more in the first sieve, 30 to 50% in the middle sieve and a maximum of 20% in the last sieve.

Sometimes the assessment was carried out on the day of ensiling, as shown in Figure 31, so it was possible to tell the producer whether it was necessary to increase or decrease the chopping size. The processing and breaking of the grains was also analysed. In order to make the most of the starch in the grain, it is necessary to at least "bruise" the grain, otherwise there is a large loss through the faeces.

When these proportions are not maintained, they can cause other digestive disorders such as abomasal displacement, as well as acidosis, a reduction in milk fat and foot changes. Excessive chopping causes a reduction in chewing and rumination time, resulting in less saliva being produced and consequently less sodium bicarbonate, resulting in a drop in pH. According to Sarashina (1989), when there is a large presence of small particles in the diet, there is greater rumen fermentation, resulting in reduced abomasal motility and an increase in the accumulation of gas in the abomasum, predisposing it to displacement.

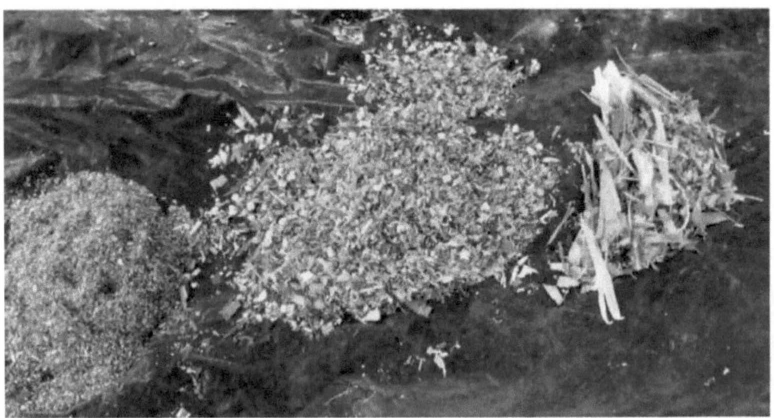

Figure 31 - Separation of maize silage using the Penn State sieve.
Source: Tomasini (2015).

4.2.3 Body condition score

The body condition score is an excellent tool for evaluating animals when it comes to reproductive management, balancing the diet and assessing BEN. Short and Adams (1988) described the use of available energy in ruminants, classifying each of the physiological states in order of importance as follows: 1) basal metabolism; 2) activity; 3) growth; 4) energy reserves; 5) pregnancy; 6) lactation; 7) additional energy reserves; 8) estrous cycles and early pregnancy, 9) surplus energy reserves. As we can see, if the animal has a negative energy balance, reproduction will be greatly compromised.

According to Overton and Smith (2010), the conception rate at the first service can be reduced by 50% when ECC decreases by more than 1.0 point during the first 60 days postpartum and the risk of a prolonged anovulatory condition (absence of oestrus) increases in animals where ECC falls below 2.75 or a condition where excessive loss of score occurs during the early postpartum period. Moreira et al. (2000), described that a CKC lower than 2.5 influences the insemination protocol, reducing the pregnancy rate and increasing costs.

On some of the farms we visited, we found cows with a body score of 2.5 or less (Figure 32). Some of the cows had this score because of their high milk production in the immediate postpartum period, while others had suffered some clinical condition, such as retained placenta. For these animals it was recommended to add ground maize to the diet in order to increase the energy in the diet and consequently the body score.

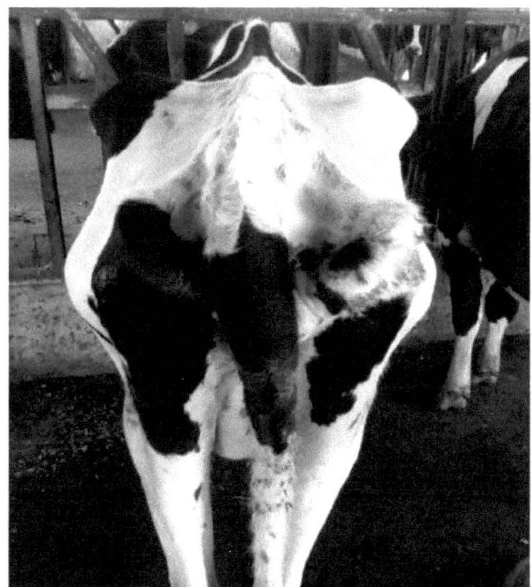
Figure 32 - Cow with body score 2.0.
Source: Tomasini (2015)

The gynaecological examination of this cow showed atrophied ovaries, with no activity, due to a decrease in the production of hypothalamic, pituitary and steroid hormones. According to Ferreira (1993), there is a minimum weight for each cow, where

below this weight, ovarian activity ceases. This occurs when there is a loss of 25 to 30 per cent of adult weight.

Evaluating the ECC in pre-calving cows is very important, because it is at this stage that problems begin, or if carried out correctly, where we find the solution to many problems. According to Kellog (2010), the ideal score for pre-calving cows is between 3.0 and 3.5. However, some cows arrive at pre-calving with a score of 4.0 or more (Figure 33), and most of the time these animals have calved later, which increases their body score because they will have a longer lactation and consequently decrease their milk production and increase their body score. Some tools can be used to correct this excess weight, including the use of bovine somatotropin (bST). BST has been used in cows that are late to calve, prolonging lactation. According to Bauman and Vernon (1993) in cows that are gaining ECC, the synthesis and deposition of lipids in adipose tissue is reduced by the action of bST, which in turn increases the availability of nutrients and their utilisation for milk production, helping to correct the body score and increasing milk production. This happens through a decrease in body fat, an increase in circulating non-esterified fatty acids (NFAs) and an increase in the percentage of fat present in milk (SECHEN et al., 1989).

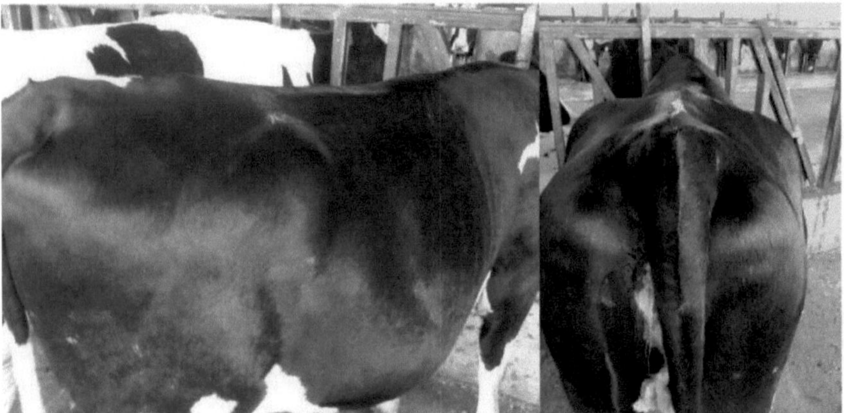

Figure 33 - Cow with ECC of 4.0. Use of bST indicated.
Source: Tomasini, 2015.

4.2.4 Trough score

The trough score is widely used in large beef cattle feedlots, but it is also very suitable for dairy cattle. As Bierman (2001) describes, the trough score is the supervision and execution to determine, in an acceptable and coherent way, the amount of food an animal can consume in a given period of time. The management of the trough represents a major challenge, as the person carrying it out must have a good understanding so as not to jeopardise the feeding of the cows.

The activities on the technical assistance properties usually lasted around two or three hours, during which time the cows stayed in the pens, where they were fed, basically maize silage and feed. It was then always assessed whether the cows were leaving leftovers in the trough or whether they were eating everything. The trough score was assessed according to Bolsen and Pollard (2004).

A score of 0 is when there are no leftovers and the trough is often licked clean (Figure 34). In the semi-extensive system, a trough score of 0 is usually found when there is a low supply of pasture, either in the transition period from one pasture to another or in times of low rainfall, so the animals reduce their consumption due to the low supply and the trough does not increase in supply. This score is also found when there is an error in the formulation of the diet or by the attendant.

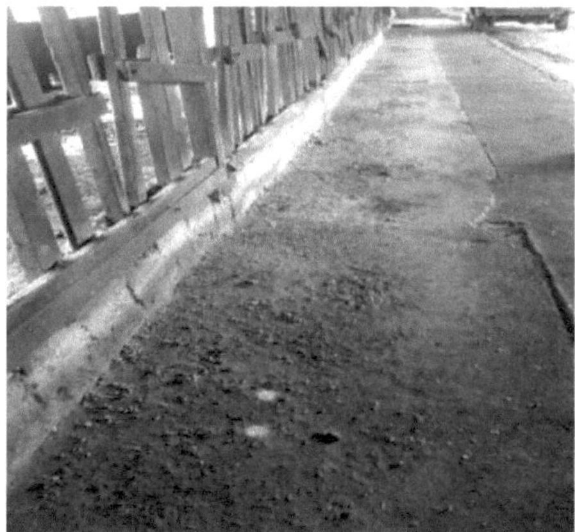
Figure 34 - Trough score 0.
Source: Tomasini (2015).

In scores 1 and 2 there is a small surplus of food, around 5% (Figure 35). This leftover is important because it shows that the animal was satisfied with its dry matter intake.

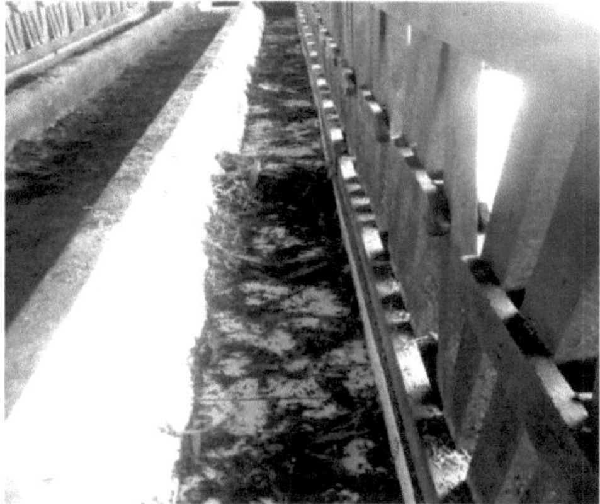
Figure 35 - Trough score 2.
Source: Tomasini (2015).

In trough score 3, the cows may be overfed or the feed may not be in good condition (Figure 36). In this case, the cows were being fed incorrectly, causing a lot of food waste and increasing costs. The trough score helps prevent this waste, in agreement with Bierman and Pritchard (1996).

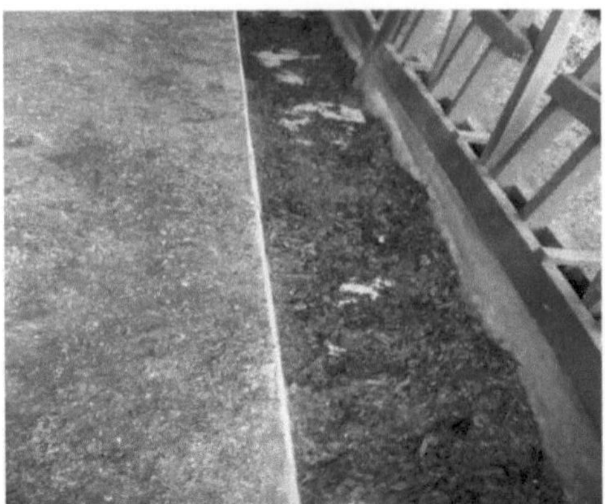

Figure 36 - Trough score 3, surplus higher than desired.
Source: Tomasini (2015).

At score 4 there is a large surplus where you should check what the problem is (Figure 37), review the amount of feed being given and make sure the cows are comfortable feeding. In summer, heat stress is related to reduced feed intake, causing problems if we don't pay attention.

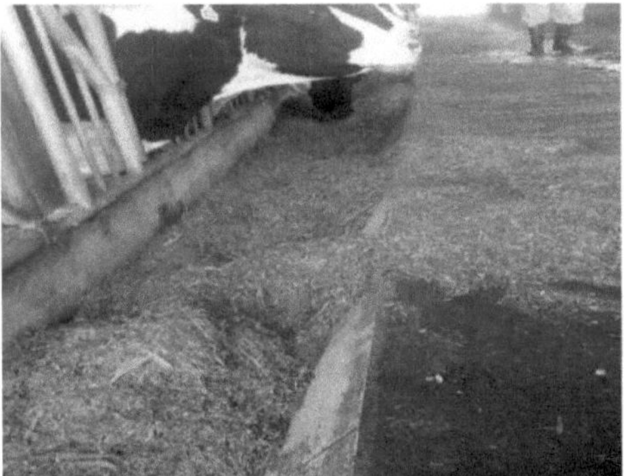

Figure 37 - Trough score 4, large quantities of feed.
Source: Tomasini (2015).

Trough score 5 means that the feed remains intact (Figure 38). Most of the time this is related to some disease, among which the most common during the internship period were parasitic sadness and non-specific pneumonia. The trough score becomes interesting at the time of clinical care, where it is observed whether the animal has eaten or not.

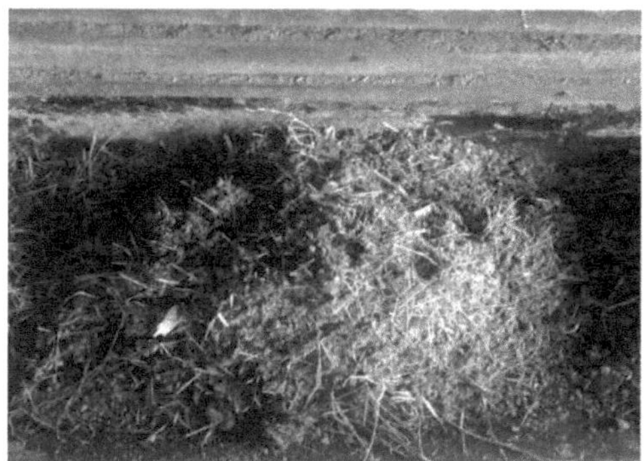
Figure 38 - Trough score 5, intact feed.
Source: Tomasini (2015).

4.2.5   Rumen score

The rumen score is a method of evaluating feed intake, but evaluating rumen filling alone is not very reliable, as there are many differences between cows. Therefore, the ideal is to evaluate and relate to the trough score, after meals and always at the same time. By making this joint assessment, it is possible to reach a reliable conclusion as to how the IMS is doing. According to Hartnell and Satter (1979), rumen fill is defined by the total amount of liquid and dry matter (kg) in the rumen, and is related to IMS, feed composition, digestibility and the rate of passage of ingested feed. Burfeind et al. (2010), found a relationship between IMS and rumen fill, however using measurements of the depth of the left paralumbar fossa (Figure 39), they detected considerable change (up to 4.8 cm) within 70 ± 5 min, which shows the great variability that is found.

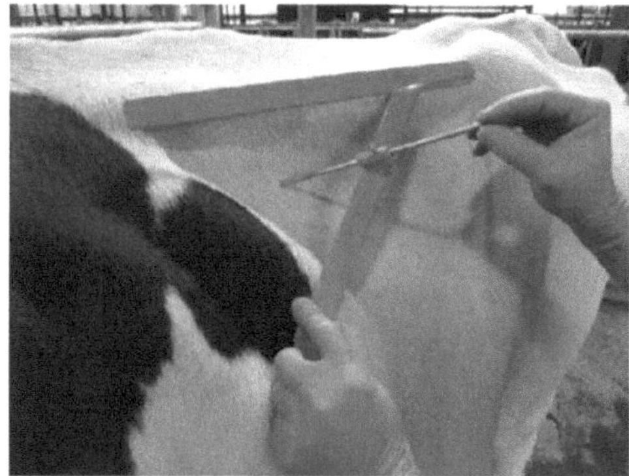
Figure 39 - Measurement of the paralumbar fossa.
Source: Burfeind et al. (2010).

Analysing rumen filling in Figure 40, we can see that feed intake was lower than necessary, as the paralumbar fossa is partially filled. Figure 41 shows greater rumen filling, which is ideal for lactating cows, according to Zaaijer and Noordhuizen (2001).

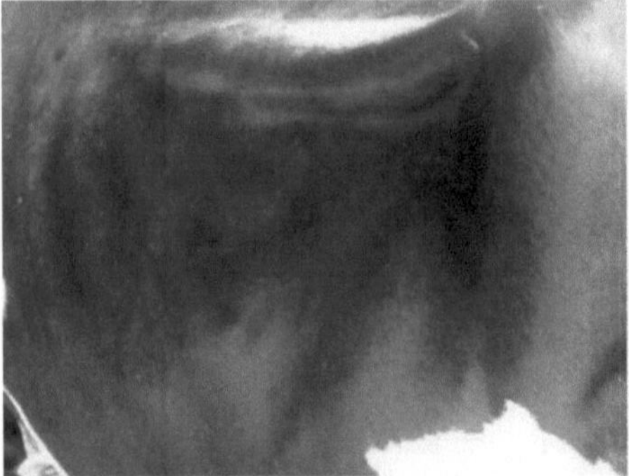

Figure 40 - Rumen score 2, low IMS.
Source: Tomasini (2015).

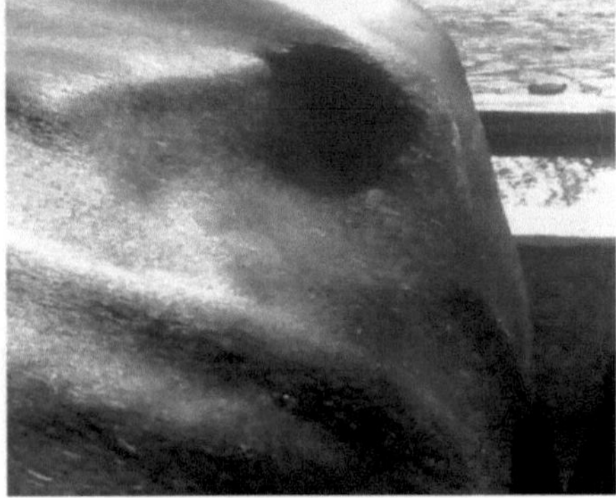

Figure 41 - Rumen score 3, ideal for lactating cows.
Source: Tomasini (2015).

CHAPTER 5

FINAL CONSIDERATIONS

The supervised curricular internship for the completion of the Veterinary Medicine course is of great importance for the student's training, because through this phase the knowledge acquired at university can be associated with practice in the field, thus developing an opinion and critical sense. In the field, you can see the importance of the Veterinarian on dairy farms, helping producers with animal management, nutrition, reproduction and disease prevention.

REFERENCES

BAUMAN, D.E., VERNON, R.G. Effects of exogenous bovine somatotropin on lactation. **Annual Review of Nutrition.** v.13, p.437-461, 1993.

BICALHO, R. C. et al. Association Between a Visual and an Automated Locomotion Score in Lactating Holstein Cows. **Journal of Dairy Science.** v. 90, No. 7, 2007.

BIERMAN, S. **Bunk management and feeding strategies.** Minnesota Cattle Feeder Report B-477, 2001.

BIERMAN, S.J., PRITCHARD R.H. Effect of feed delivery management on yearling steer performance. South Dakota **Agricultural Experiment Station. Beef Report CATTLE** 96-5:17-22. 1996.

BOLSEN K. K., POLLARD G. V. Feed Bunk Management to Maximise Feed Intake. **Advances in Dairy Technology.** v. 16, p. 227, 2004.

BRENT, B. E. Relationship of acidosis to other feedlot ailments. **Journal of Animal Science.** v. 43, 1976.

BURFEIND O. et al. Technical note: evaluation of a scoring system for rumen fill. **Journal of Dairy Science.** v. 93 No. 8, 2010

DECHOW C.D. et al. Correlations among body condition scores from various sources, dairy form, and cow health from the United States and Denmark. **Journal of Dairy Science.** v. 87, No. 10, 2004.

DEMBELE I. Factors contributing to the incidence and prevalence of lameness on Czech dairy farms. **Journal of Animal Science.** v. 51, p. 102-109, 2006.

EDMONSON A.J. et al. A Body Condition Scoring Chart for Holstein Dairy Cows. **Journal of Dairy Science,** v. 72: p. 68-78, 1989.

ESPEJO L.A., ENDRES M.I., SALFER J.A. Prevalence of Lameness in High- Producing Holstein Cows Housed in Freestall Barns in Minnesota. **Journal of Dairy Science,** v. 89 No. 8, 2006.

FERREIRA, A. M. Nutrition and Ovarian Activity in Cattle: A review. **Pesquisa Agropecuária Brasileira, Brasília**, v 28, n 9, p. 1077-1093, 1993.

FERREIRA, M. C. N. et al. **Impact of body condition on the pregnancy rate of Nelore cows grazing under a fixed-time artificial insemination (FTAI) programme.** Semina: Ciências Agrárias, Londrina, v. 34, n. 4, p. 1861-1868. 2013.

FLOWER, F.C., WEARY, D.M. **Gait assessment in dairy cattle**. The Animal Consortium, p. 87-95, 2008.

GARLEB, K. A., et al. Chemical composition and digestibility of fibre fractions of certain by-products feeds tuffs fed to ruminal. Journal Animal Science. v. 66, p. 2650-2660, 1988.

GONZÁLEZ, F.H.D, DURR, J.W, FONTANELI, R.S. Using milk to monitor the nutrition and metabolism of dairy cows. Porto Alegre - RS, Brazil, 2001.

GREENOUGH, P. R. Bovine Laminitis and Lameness. Saunders Elsevier, 2007.

HARTNELL, G. F., SATTER, L. D. Determination of rumen fill, retention time and ruminal turnover rates of ingesta at different stages of lactation in dairy cows. Journal of Animal Science, v. 48, No. 2, 1979.

HEINRICHS, J.; KONONOFF, P. J. Evaluating particle size of forages and TMRs using the New Penn State Forage Particle Separator. Pennsylvania State University, College of Agricultural Sciences, Cooperative Extension DAS 02-42. 2002.

HULSEN J. Cow Signals - A practical guide for dairy farm management. 2007.

HUSSEIN, M. et al. Conjugated linoleic acid-induced milk fat depression in lactating ewes is accompanied by reduced expression of mammary genes involved in lipid synthesis. Journal of Dairy Science, v. 96 No. 6, 2013.

HUTJENS, M.F. Manureology 101. Four-State Dairy Nutrition & Management Conference Proceedings. p. 59-61. 2010.

IBGE, Directorate of Research, Agricultural Coordination, Quarterly Milk Survey. Mar. 2015.

JÚNIOR, G.N., SANTOS, E.B. Evolution of milk production in Brazil. Veterinary and Zootechnical Journal. 2013.

JUAREZ, S.T., ROBINSON P.H. Locomotion Scoring Your Cows: Use and Interpretation. Department of Animal Science University of California, Davis. 2002.

JUAREZ, S.T. et al. Impact of lameness on behaviour and productivity of lactating Holstein cows. Applied Animal Behaviour Science. v. 83, p. 1-14, 2003.

KELLOGG, W. Body Condition Scoring with Dairy Cattle. Cooperative Extension Service, University of Arkansas, U.S. Department of Agriculture, and county governments cooperating, 2010.

LAMMERS, B.P.; BUCKMASTER, D.R.; HEINRICHS, A.J. A simple method for the analysis of particle sizes of forage and total mixed rations. Journal of Dairy Science, v.79, p. 922-928, 1996.

LOY, D. Feed bunk management. Extension Beef Specialist, Iowa State University. 1997.

LEE, L.A., FERGUSON, J.D., GALLIGAN D.T. Effect of Disease on Days Open Assessed by Survival Analysis. Journal of Dairy Science v. 72, No. 4, 1989.

MELENDEZ, P. et al. The association between lameness, ovarian cysts and fertility in lactating dairy cows. Theriogenology. v. 59, p. 927-937, 2003.

MOREIRA, et al. Effect of Body Condition on Reproductive Efficiency of Lactating Dairy Cows Receiving a Timed Insemination. Theriogenology. v. 53: p. 1305-1319, 2000.

MUHLBACH, P.R.F. et al. Nutritional aspects that affect milk quality. In: UFRGS ANNUAL MEETING ON RUMINANT NUTRITION, 2, 2000. Porto Alegre. Proceedings... Porto Alegre: UFRGS Department of Animal Science, p. 73-102, 2000.

MURRAY R.D. Epidemiology of lameness in dairy cattle: Description and analysis of foot lesions. Veterinary Record. v. 138, p. 586-591. 1996.

NAIBO, W. Disposal factors in dairy cows in the western region of Santa Catarina. Anais...Xanxerê: V Mostra Universitária, 2014.

NOCEK, J. E. Bovine acidosis: implications in laminitis. Journal of Dairy Science, Champaign. v. 80, n. 5, p. 1005-1028, 1997.

NORDLUND, K. V. et al. Investigation Strategies for Laminitis Problem Herds. Journal of Dairy Science. v. 87, E. Suppl., 2004

OLECHNOWICZ J., JAÔKOWSKI J. M. Body condition related to lameness in dairy cows. Institute of Veterinary Medicine, Faculty of Animal Breeding and Biology, Poznan University of Life Sciences, Wolynska. v. 35, p. 60-637 Poznaií, Poland.

OLIVEIRA, M.A., SOARES, S.R.V. How to use the Locomotion Score to monitor the health of a herd's hooves. Technical Articles - Rehagro, 2007.

OVERTON, M.W., I.J. SMITH. The Use of Records to Evaluate and Improve Transition Cow Performance. Four-State Dairy Nutrition & Management Conference Proceedings, p. 43-49, 2010.

ROSELER, D. K. et al. Development and evaluation of equations for prediction of feed intake for lactating Holstein dairy cows. Journal Dairy Science. v. 80: p. 878893, 1997.

SANTOS, G.T., CAVALIERI, F.L.B., DAMASCENO, J.C. Manejo da vaca leiteira no período transição e início da lactação. Proceedings of the II Sul-Leite: Symposium on the Sustainability of Dairy Farming in the Southern Region of Brazil. Maringá, v. 1, p. 143165, 2002.

SCHLAGETER-TELLO, A. et al. Manual and automatic locomotion scoring systems in dairy cows: A review. Preventive Veterinary Medicine, v. 116, p. 12-25, 2014.

SECHEN, S.J. et al. Effect of somatotropin on kinetics of nonesterified fatty acids and partition of energy, carbon and nitrogen in lactating dairy cows. Journal of Dairy Science. v.72, n.1, p.57-59, 1989.

SHORT, R.E., ADAMS, D.C. Nutritional and hormonal interrelationships in beef cattle reproduction. Canadian Journal of Animal Science, v.68, p.29, 1988.

SPRECHER D.J., HOSTETLER D.E., KANEENE J.B. A lameness scoring system that uses posture and gait to predict dairy cattle reproductive performance. Theriogenology, v. 47, p. 1179-1187, 1997.

STALLINGS, C.C., 1993. Manure Scoring as a Management Tool. Department of Dairy Science, Virginia Tech, Blacksburg, VA 24061-0315 U.S.A. 1993.

STOKES, et al. Managing Milk Composition: Evaluating Herd Potential. Texas A&M Agrilife Extension, 2000.

SULAYEMAN M., FROMSA A. Lameness in Dairy Cattle: Prevalence, Risk Factors and Impact on Milk Production. Global Veterinaria. v. 8 (1): p. 01-07, 2012.

TIBRU, I. Quantification of feeding and digestion in cows. Lucrâri Stiintifice Medicina Veterinarã. v. XLIII (2), 2010, Timiçoara.

WARNICK L.D. et al. The Effect of Lameness on Milk Production in Dairy Cows. Journal of Dairy Science v. 84, No. 9, 2001.

WILDMAN E. E. et al. A dairy cow body condition scoring system and its relationship to selected production characteristics. Journal of Dairy Science, v. 65, p. 495-501, 1982.

ZAAIJER, D.; NOORDHUIZEN, J.P.T.M. Dairy cow monitoring in relation to fertility performance. Irish Veterinary Journal, 2001.

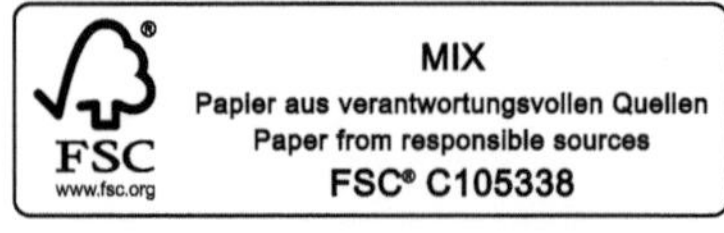

Printed by Books on Demand GmbH, Norderstedt / Germany